T0413193

Phlebotomy Fundamentals

Phlebotomy Fundamentals

Anthony Raia

Rev. date: 08/28/2019

To order additional copies of this book, contact:
Xlibris
1-888-795-4274
www.Xlibris.com
Orders@Xlibris.com
786187

CONTENTS

Acknowledgement

I would like to thank the following for their help and support in the making of this text book beginning with my publisher Xlibris publishing. Your staff has been exceptional, from the editing to marketing to helping with the set up of the website and cover of the book. Next is my wonderful wife, Lori, thank you for inspiring me and doing some proof reading amongst all of the other things you were doing such as taking the kids to school, and homework and games, thank you. Also involved in the making of the book are the providers from Beth Israel Deaconess Medical center. Dr. Li Zhou, Dr. Kelly Ford, Dr. James Heckman, and Dr. Angela Fowler Brown. Thank you for taking the time during your busy schedules to proof read the body systems and to check for accuracy. The journey to making the book also included filming phlebotomy, EKG, and vitals for students to view. This could not have been possible without the help from Tom laws, Tom, thank you for taking the time to set up all your equipment and endless hours of filming. To Mike Barthe, Matilda Ganjolli, Natalie Colon, Linda Macmillan, and Fantastic Remy (yes, his name is Fantastic), thank you for volunteering your time in the making of the video. To my cousin Cathy and her husband Jesse, thank you for taking interest in the book and taking time to read and give your opinion, it was a great help during the process. To Heather Wathey, from the very beginning when book only had a few pages you helped in proof reading and consistantly made sure I stayed on track until it's completion. Thank you Heather. And to Whitney Griesbach, you too, took great interest in the making of the book by reviewing it's contents and give some ideas that would make the book more informative. To Kevin Murphy, thank you for taking the time to proof read and make corrections where necessary in the begininning phase of the book. And to my friends who supported me; Jackie Ruggiero, Joe Santoro, Ed and Tara Herries, Ann Archer, and Julie Foiadelli. Thank you all.

Best,
Anthony Raia

Chapter 1

The Past and Present

From the early days, blood has been a miracle substance. Hippocrates (460-377 BC) believed that removing foreign substances from the blood would put the person back into a normal state. The technique used was phlebotomy. The term phlebotomy means bloodletting and is broken down into two parts from the Greek words, **phlebos** and **tomy.** "Phlebo" means veins "tomy" means incision. Together they mean an incision into a vein to remove blood. Some thought that by using a sharp instrument to cut into a vein that this would cleanse the body of evil spirits. Around the year 1210 barber surgeons were formed, yes you read this correctly, barbers. Soon after, barbers and surgeons duties were divided. To signify this, barbers wore short robes while surgeons wore long robes and by doing this barbers were now forbidden to perform any type of surgery with the exception of bloodletting (phlebotomy). The barber also extracted teeth, cupping, leeching, administer enema's and some minor wound surgery. The barber placed a striped red, white, and blue pole outside of his place of business. The pole represents; red for blood, blue for veins, and white for bandages. In fact, to this day, outside some barber shops you may see a red white and blue pole. By the 19th century, barbers were discouraged to perform bloodletting by surgeons because many surgeons felt it posed a danger to people. Eventually it became law that barbers were not permitted to perform any type of bloodletting or surgical procedure.

Important Dates in Phlebotomy

- 1210 Barber surgeons formed.
- 1400 BC Egyptian paintings on tombs depicting leeches in patients to remove blood.
- 1799 Possible contribution to George Washington's death after being bled four times in two days.
- 1800 Brass syringes attached to a cup for bloodletting.
- 1900 Barber surgeons disbanded.

Modern Day Phlebotomy

Today's phlebotomist has a wide range of responsibilities including:

- Perform venous punctures (Drawing blood from a vein)
- Capillary punctures (Finger sticks)
- Prepare specimens for collection and proper labeling of tubes collected
- Perform glucose tests (using a glucometer)
- Collect urine samples and perform dip stick test
- Document specimen results
- Transport properly labeled specimens to lab or prepare specimens for pick-up
- Perform quality control checks
- Perform vitals (Blood pressure, pulse, respiration, temperature, and O2 saturation)
- Perform Electrocardiography (EKG)
- Maintain safe working conditions
- Promote public relations fo both staff and paients
- Participate in continuing education programs (this will allow you to comply with updated and revised procedures)

Professionalism

As in any industry, practicing professionalism defines the qualities and characteristic of an individual. You may have heard that the first impression is the most important. This is very true. It does not matter how good a healthcare provider you are, if you lack professionalism you will be viewed as such. I have been to many practices sometimes as a patient, and it disturbs me when my name is called and the healthcare worker will say come in and have a seat. What's wrong with this? I'll tell you. Where is, Hi my name is? And most importantly, when possible, a hand shake and looking into their eyes? I guarantee you, if you call them by name (usually their last name) then saying hello my name is, along with a hand shake, well at first they may look at you like you had two heads, but most importantly you will have characterized yourself as a professional. Professionalism also includes your work ethics, speaking habits, and overall appearance. A professional phlebotomist, or any healthcare worker should always exhibit the following: Integrity, Motivation, Dependability, and will always be sensitive to the patients needs and wants and always shows compassion. Let's now talk about these important characteristics individually.

Integrity: Integrity is referred to as honesty and is probably what I would call the foundation. This is making sure you have the correct patient, correct tubes, and following laboratory protocol and procedures. Mistakes can occur. For instance you drew two lavender top tubes instead of one lavender and one serum separator tube. Reporting this mistake to your lab supervisor or better yet, notify the patient before he leaves the lab shows you have owned up to your mistake and correct it swiftly. Remember, you are the backbone of the field. The doctors and nurses most importantly, the patient rely on your utmost attention.

Motivation: I believe motivation comes from within a person. Nobody can give you motivation. Willing to take on a new task, working at your maximum each and every day, not complaining, but rather, finding and sharing solutions will make the overall working environment more pleasurable and will decrease errors. Remember motivation is the vehicle which will drive you to being successful. It also shows your attitude towards life.

Dependability: Dependability coincides with motivation. When a person is motivated they will also be dependable. Dependability means arriving to work on time, multi-tasking, assisting a co-worker, these are just to mention a few. Please do not in any way use motivation or dependability as a monetary vehicle. It will become your nemesis and will take away your drive to focus on what really matters. "The patient".

Sensitivity and Compassion: like motivation and dependability, sensitivity and compassion coinside with each other. This means understanding the patient's needs and wants. This refers to whether a patient is coming in for a yearly check-up or simply just not feeling well. For example, a patient makes an appointment with the doctor. You perform a blood pressure and the blood pressure seems high. You report this to the doctor or nurse prior to them seeing the patient. By doing so, this may cause the doctor to order some blood tests. Your sensitivity and compassion to alert the doctor of the high blood pressure reading shows your compassion for the patients well-being.

Chapter 2

The History of Laboratory Administration

Before beginning to explore the different departments in a laboratory and their functions, let's begin with the CLIA act of 1988. CLIA stands for Clinical Laboratory Improvement Amendment. The CLIA act was signed on October 31, 1988 and went into effect in 1992. What this means is that every laboratory regardless of size or location must successfully pass a compliance inspection before receiving a certificate of compliance. The certificate signifies to the patient that all equipment used to collect and test specimens are in compliance and that all laboratory results are accurate. Now let's look at the various departments of a laboratory and some of the common tests performed along with the collection tube used and the number of inversions.

As mentioned, laboratories are divided and sub-divided into functional working sections. They are; Hematology, Chemistry, Microbiology, Blood bank, Immunology, Serology. Some larger laboratories may perform tissue biopsy's either after surgery or autopsy. I suggest that you become familiar with the various departments in your oranization. This will help you understand and appreciate the role of each department. Let's now discuss in detail each department and the most common tests performed individually.

Hematology Lab: Hematology is the study of blood. The most commonly used tube in hematology is the lavender top tube. After obtaining a blood sample the tube is inverted 8-10 times gently to mix the anticoagulant in the tube with the blood. Do not shake the tube as this will cause hemolysis (destruction of red blood cells). The hematology department performs the following tests.

Complete Blood Count (CBC): A complete blood count covers the following tests.

Red Blood Cell Count (RBC) also known as an erythrocyte count. This identifies the percentage of red blood cells (erythrocytes) in a volume of whole blood. Red blood cells are the most common cell and their count is in the millions.

Hemoglobin (Hgb): Hemoglobin is a protein within a red blood cell that carries oxygen to the organs and gives blood it's red color.

Hematocrit (HCT): Hematocrit is the percentage of red blood cells to the volume of whole blood plus many other RBC indices.

Platelet count: The role of a platelet is blood clotting. When a platelet count is low or higher than normal this may be an indication of a potential bleeding disorder.

White Blood Cell Count (WBC) also referred to as a leukocyte count. This determines the number of white blood cells in a volume of blood.

White blood cell differential count (CBC with diff) This test evalutes the following cells, their shape and size.

Granulocyte: There are three types of granulocytes. Neutrophil, Eosinophil, and Basophil. The best way to remember them is they are known as the phil brothers. First let's begin with neutrophils. 65% of the white blood cells are neutrophils. Neutrophil counts rise when a bacterial infection occurs. The total life span of a neutrophil is six hours to a few day's. Next we have eosinophils. Approximately 3% of the white blood cells are eosinophils. They engulf and detoxify foreign protein and rise in number with allergies and when parasite infections occur. The total life span of an eosinophil is eight to twelve days. Last we have basophils. Approximately 1% or less of the white blood cell count are basophils. They help in the inflammatory response by releasing histamine and heparin.

Chemistry Department: The chemistry department is typically the largest department and receives the most blood samples, and depending on the tests, the following tube types are collected. Red top tube (contains no additive), Serum Separator tube (SST). The SST tube contains a separator gel. Do not shake the tube as this will cause hemolysis. If you are responsible for centrifuging the specimen, the tube should be placed in a tube holder standing erect for thirty minutes to allow clotting and then centriguged for fifteen minutes. Let's now review some of the most common tests performed pertaining to each vital organ and body system.

Adrenal Glands
- Cortisol: Cortisol is the primary glucocorticoid and is secreted by the adrenal cortex in response to ACTH (adrenocorticotropic hormone). ACTH helps metabolize nutrients and regulate the immune system. Cortisol levels are ordered when signs of adrenal dysfunction is suspected. Blood tests confirming a high level of cortsol indicates adrenal hyperfunction (Cushing's Syndrome). Blood tests confirming decreased levels of cortisol indicates adrenal hypofunction (Addison's disease).

Skeletal System
- **Calcium:** The body absorbes calcium from the gastrointestinal tract, this is however, sufficient amount of vitamin D is present. 98% of calcium is found in the bones and teeth. When calcium levels fall below the normal range calcium ions may shift from the bones and teeth to maintain blood levels. Increased levels

of serum calcium (Hypercalcemia) may indicate the following. Hyperparathyroidism, multiple myeloma, metastatic carcinoma, multiple fractures, insufficient calcium secretion, prolonged immobilization, excessive calcium intake such as overuse of antacids.

Decreased levels of serum calcium (hypocalcemia) may indicate the following. Renal failure, malabsorption, hypoparathyroidism, acute pancreatitis, Cushing's Syndrome, peritonitis.

Central Nervous System (C N S)

- Lithium: Lithium levels are performed to evaluate and to help avoid toxic levels and to avoid renal damage.

Heart

- **Cholesterol:** Cholesterol is a component found in the cell membrane and lipoproteins and is absorbed from diet and is broken down in the liver as well as some body tissues. A diet which includes a high saturated intake of fat can raise cholesterol levels which stimulates absorption of lipids.

  Increased levels of serum cholesterol (hypercholesterolemia) may indcate risk of coronary artery disease, pancreatitis, bile duct blockage, hypothyroidism.

  Decreased levels of serum cholesterol (hypocholesterolemia) may indicate malnutrition, hyperthyroidism.

- **Triglycerides:** Triglycerides are the primary storage of lipids which also contitutes 95% of fatty tissue.

  Increased serum triglycerideds may indcate risk of coronary artery disease (CAD), overconsumption of alcohol, diabetes.

Decreased serum triglycerides may indcate Malnutrition.

Kidney

- Magnesium: Magnesium is an electrolyte which helps regulate intracelluar metabolism. Magnesium also initiates several essential enzymes as well as aiding the transport of sodium and potassium across cell membranes. Magnesium is absorped In the small intestine and is excreted in urine and feces.

- **Creatinine:** Creatinine is formed in the kidney, liver, pancreas, and small intestine mucosa and is an end product of protein.

  Increased serum creatnine levels may indicate pregnancy, hyperthyroidism, excessive intake in dietary protein.

- Uric Acid: Uric acid clears the body by glomerular filtration. However, it is important to know that uric acid is not very soluble. Uric acid levels may also increase with starvaton, high purine diet, abuse of alcohol.

- Blood Urea Nitrogen (BUN): The principal end product of protein metabolism is the nitrogen portion of urea. Urea is formed in the liver from ammonia and excreted by the kidneys. Blood urea nitrogen is ordered to evaluate renal function and to detect renal disease.

  Increased blood urea nitrogen may indicate, urinary tract obstructon, renal disease, reduced renal blood flow such as in dehydration.

  Decreased blood urea nitrogen may indicate, malnutrition, severe hepatiic damage, overhydration.

Liver

- Alanine aminotransferase (ALT): Alanine aninotransferase aslo known as serum glutamic-pyruvic (SGPT) is necessary for tissue energy production. Often times before jaundice appears which causes extremely high serum levels, SGPT/ALT is released from the cytoplasm into the bloodstream.

  High levels of SGPT/ALT may indicate, drug induced hepatitis, hepatic disease.

  Moderate to high levels of SGPT/ALT may indicate, cholecystitis, chronic hepatitis, hepatic congestion due to heart failure.

  Moderate to slight levels of SGPT/ALT may indicate, acute cirrhosis, drug induced alcoholic hepatitis.

- Alpha-fetoprotein (AFP): A glycoprotein, alpha-fetoprotein is produced by fetal tissue during fetal development. After 14 week gestation the levels of AFP rise sharply, by as much as 90% On occasion, nonpregnant patients may experience high levels of AFP with cancer of the pancreas, stomach.

  Slightly high levels of AFP in nonpregnant patients may indicate, alcholic cirrhosis, chronic or acute hepatitis.

  High levels of AFP after 14 weeks gestation may indicate, spina bifida, intrauterine death.

- Ammonia: Ammonia is a nonprotein nitrogen compound which is absorbed in the intestinal tract and helps maintain acid base balance. Generally the nitrogen portion of ammonia is to aid in rebuilding amino acids; afterwords, ammonia is converted into urea in the liver for excretion by the kidneys. Ammonia can bypass the liver in diseases such as cirrhosis of the liver.

High levels of ammonia may indicate, gastrointestinal hemorrhage, severe congestive heart failure.

- Total Bilirubin: Total Bilirubin is a breakdown product of hemoglobin. Bound to albumin, bilirubin is transported to the liver and mixed with glucuronide. Afterwords, bilirubin is excreted in the bile. During biliary obstruction, bilirubin is obstructed from it's normal flow through the liver causing bilirubin to overflow into the bloodstream. This leads to jaundice.

Increased serum indirect bilirubin may indicate, hepatic damage, hemolytic anemia.

Increased serum direct bilirubin may indicate, biliary obstruction.

Increased direct and indirect bilirubin may indicate, biliary obstruction with hepatic obstruction, prolonged hemolysis.

- Vitamin B12 and folate: Vitamin B12 is a water soluble vitamin which contains cobalt (an element found in the liver). Vitamin B12 is absorbed in the ileum and stored in the liver. Like vitamin B12, folate (folic acid) is water soluble. The body stores a small amount of folic acid in the liver.

Increased levels of serum folic acid (folate) may indicate, overconsumption of dietary folic acid suppliments.

Increased levels of serum B12 may indicate, hepatic damage, overconsumption of dietary supplements.

Decreased levels of serum folic acid (folate) may indicate, anemia, leukopenia, pregnancy, thrombocytopenia, chronic alcoholism, insufficient dietary intake.

Decreased levels of serum vitamin B12 may indicate, pregnancy, insufficient intake of vitamin B12 (common in patients who are strict vegetarians), malabsorption of vitamin B12.

Pancreas

- Glucose: Glucose is the main source of energy and comes from foods containing carbohydrates. Upon consumption of food the hormone insuline is released into the blood stream as the levels of glucose increases. If blood glucose levels remain high damage to the kidneys, eyes, nerves, and blood vessels can occur.
- Lipase: Lipase is produced in the pancreas and secreted into the duodenum. Lipase converts triglycerides and fats into fatty acids and glycerol.

Increased levels of lipase may indicate, pancreatic duct obstruction, acute pancreatitis, pancreatic cancer, renal disease.

Prostate

- Acid phosphatase: Acid phosphatase is made up of a group of phosphatase enzymes and appears mainly in the prostate and semen. Small amounts of acid phosphatase is also found in the spleen, liver, bone marrow, red blood cells, and platelets.

Increased levels of acid phosphatase may indicate a tumor has spread in the prostate, prostatic infarction, multiple myeloma.

- Prostate specific antigen (PSA): The PSA is a protein produced by the prostate gland. An elevation of PSA levels may indicate a non-cancerous condition such as prosatitis, Benign Prostatic Hyperplasia (BPH), or it may indicate prostate cancer.

Liver

- Alkaline phosphatase (ALP): Alkaline phosphatase aids in bone calcification and lipid transport.

  Increased alkaline phosphatase levels may indicate, hyperparathyroidism, biliary obstruction, bone metastasis.

  Moderate increase of alkaline phosphatase levels may indicate, viral hepatitis, cirrhosis of the liver, mononucleosis.

Liver or Heart

- Aspartate aminotransferase (AST): Aspartate aminotransferase also known as serum glutamic oxaloacetic transaminase (SGOT) is an enzyme found in the cells of the liver, skeletal muscles, kidneys, heart, and pancreas.

  Extremely high levels of AST/SGOT may indicate, severe skeletal muscle trauma, acute viral hepatitis, drug-induced hepatic injury.

  High levels of AST/SGOT may indicate, alcoholic cirrhosis, myocardial infarction (MI), severe infectious mononucleosis.:

  Moderate to high levels of AST/SGOT may indicate, chronic hepatisis.

  Slight to moderate levels of AST/SGOT may indicate, acute pancreatitis, fatty liver, pulmonary emboli, biliary obstruction.

Prostate and Liver

- Amylase: Amylase Is found in the salivary glands and the pancreas ans is secreted into the gastrointestinal tract which helps digest starch and glycogen in the stomach, mouth and intestine.

Increased levels of amylase may indicate, acute pancreatitis.

Moderate levels of amylase may indicate, pancreatic cancer, obstruction of the common bile duct or pancreatic duct.

Decreased level of amylase may indicate, hepatisis, cirrhosis, pancreatic cancer, chronic pancreatitis, toxemia of pregnancy.

Heart or Muscle

- Creatine kinase (CK): Also know as creatine phosphokinase (CPK) is an enzyme which has a important role in energy production.

Increased creatine kinase levels may indicate, carbone monoxide poisoning, muscle damage such as myocardial infarction (heart attack), muscular dystrophy, hypothyroidism.

Heart, Kidney, Adrenal glands

- Electrolytes (Sodium, potassium, chloride): Sodium helps maintain acid balance as well as influences potassium and chloride levels. Sodium is absorbed in the intestines and excreted by the kidneys.

increased sodium levels (hypernatremia) may be caused by excessive sodium intake or inadequate water intake such as severe vomiting, severe diarrhea, diabetes insipidus.

Decreased sodium levels (hyponatremia) may be caused by inadequate sodium intake, excessive sodium loss such as diarrhea, profuse sweating, vomiting, diuretic therapy.

Potassium

- Potassium maintains equalibrium as well as helps regulate muscle activity and is also important in maintaining electrical conduction within the skeletal and cardiac muscles. Potassium is also important iin regulating acid base balance and aids in kidney function.

  Increased levels of potassium (hyperkalemia) may be an indication of, renal failure, myocardial infarction(heart attack), addison's disease.

  Decreased leves of potassium (hypokalemia) may be an indication of loss of body fluids, Cushing's syndrome, excessive licorice intake

Chloride

- Chloride is absorbed in from the intestines and excreted from the kidneys. Chloride helps regulate blood volume and arterial blood pressure.

  Increased levels of chloride (hyperchloremia) may be an indication of, severe hydration, renal failure (shut down).

  Decreased levels of chloride (hypochloremia) may be an indication of, Addison's disease, excessive vomiting, chronic renal failure.

Other tests performed in the chemistry lab are:

Endocrine lab:

- Thyroid Stimulating Hormone (TSH): This test is performed to detect hypothyroidism (underactive thyroid) or hyperthyroidism (Graves disease).

- Human Chroionic Gonadotropin (HCG): The primary purpose of an HCG test us used to detect early pregnancy. The secondary purpose is used to detect ectopic pregnancy (tubal pregnancy).

- Follicle Stimulating Hormone (FSH): The primary purpose of this test is to detect infertility, and disorders of the menstrual cycle.

- Fasting Blood Sugar (FBS): The purpose of an FBS is used in detecting diabetes mellitis. Take note, when an FBS is ordered the patient should be instructed to fast) nothing by mouth for at least eight hours prior to the test. This will ensure the accuracy of the test.

- Glucose tolerance test (GTT): The purpose of this test is to evaluate how the body responds to a high volume of known glucose intake. Just as a fasting blood sugar, the patient needs to fast for at least eight hours prior to the test for acccurate baseline results. Prior to the test, the patient should be asked if he/she has had anything to eat or drink. If the patient consumed food or beverage (other than water) the patient should be rescheduled. The reason is the glucose level will be invalid. If the patient has fasted begin the test. First obtain a urine sample and perform a dipstick test to ensure there is no sugar in the urine. If the urine tests positive for glucose discontinue the test and report the findings to the provider. Upon a successful urine test continue with the first blood sample by obtaining a grey top tube. Afterwords, instruct he patient to drink a specified amount of glucose drink. The drink must consumed with five minutes. The patient should also be instructed not to leave the facility during the test. After consumption of the drink, note the time and obtain blood in a grey top tube every hour for the specified amount of hours. If the patient at anytime during the test complains of nausea or vomiting, of faint (syncope), immediately notify an RN or medical staff and remain with the patient and monitor the blood pressure until help arrives.

The Chemistry Department also performs panel tests. A panel is a combination of organ specific tests. (ie; Liver function test (LFT), Cardiac enzymes).

Basic Metabolic Panel (BMP): A basic metabolic panel tests is a group of tests and is used to evaluate blood sugar levels, blood acid/base balance, kidney function. Prior to performing a BMT, the patient should fast at least eight hours prior to the test. This is to ensure accurate results. The following tests are included in a BMT. Serum sodium, serum chloride, glucose, serum posassium, BUN (blood urea nitrogen), creatinine, carbon dioxide (CO_2).

Comprehensive Metabolic Panel (CMP):
A comprehensive metabolic panel (CMP) is a group of tests which gives a detailed look of the body's metabolism and chemical balance called homeostasis. A CMP is used to detect how well the liver and kidney's are functioning, aw well as checking potassium levels, glucose levels, sodium levels, protein levels, calcium and cholesterol levels. Prior to the test the patient should fast for at least eight hours.

Immunology/ Serology Department
The Immunology/ Serology lab studies antibodies (proteins) produced by white blood cells in response to an antigen (foreign protein in the body). The Immunology/Serology department also studies and

investigates problems with the immune system. For example, an autoimmune disease. An autoimmune disease is when the body turns against it's own tissue; another example is an immunodeficiency disorder. An immunodeficiency disorder is when the body's immune system is invaded by foreign cells. An example of an immunodeficiency disorder is the Human Immunodeficiency Virus (HIV) which results in aquired immunodeficiency syndrome (AIDS). Another responsibility of the immunology/ serology department is to evaluate and determine tissue, organ, and fluid compatibility. Some of the most common tests performed are; Antinuclear Antibody (ANA), Chlamydia antibody panel, Epstein-Barr virus, Hepatitus B surface antibody (Hbs/Ab), Hepatitis B surface antigen (HbsAG), Human Immunodeficiency Virus (HIV), Rheumatoid Arthritis (RA).

Blood/Immunohematology Lab (Blood Transfusion Service)

The Blood/Immunohematology department is responsible for blood products being used for transfusions. Let us now explore each component and their role.

Red Blood Cells (Erythrocyte): Red blood cells carry oxygen to the tissues in the body and carbon dioxide away. The most commonly used purpose for transfusing red blood cells is to treat anemia.

White Blood Cells (Leukocytes):   White blood cells help fight infection and aid in the immune process.

Platelets: Platlets function in blood clot formation. Platelets are commonly used in transfusions to treat leukemia as well as other types of cancer.

Plasma: Plasma is the watery, liquid portion of the blood. It's purpose is to carry the many components of the blood through the blood stream. Plasma has several other functions such as, to help maintain blood pressure as well as help balance the levels of sodium and potassium and provides proteins to aid in blood clotting.

Type and Antibody screen: The purpose of a type and antibody screen is to determine if a person in need of a transfusion receives blood or blood products match his or her blood type. During prenatal care, mothers are typed to aid in diagnosis as well as the prevention of hemolytic disease of a newborn (HDN). HDN is a type of anemia known as erythroblastosis fetalis and occurs when the baby's blood type is positive and the mothers type is negative. Babies whose blood type are different from the mothers ar at risk of HDN>

Type and Cross Match: Typing is required to determine if a person receiving a blood transfusion matches the donors blood type. Typing is a test used to determine which of the four blood groups a person falls into. The blood groups and percentages according to the Blood Transfusion Service is as follows.

Type O	Positive	39%	Type O	Negative	9%
Type A	Positive	31%	Type A	Negative	6%
Type B	Positive	9%	Type B	Negative	2%
Type AB	Positive	3%	Type AB	Negative	1%

Upon determining a patient's blood type and group, a compatibility test known as a cross match is performed. A cross match is performed to insure that the donor's red blood cells will not react with the recipient's blood serum. Therefore, confirming the patients's identity by checking the name and date of birth is extremely important. The tube collected for a type and screen or cross match is typically a red or pink top tube.

Microbiology Lab
The Microbiology Department identifies various types of organisms such as bacteria, fungi, viruses, and parasites. For example when a patient exhibits a fever of unknown origin, the doctor may order a

blood culture (BC). Blood cultures are collected in sterile vials and are collected in pairs. Each vial contains a thioglycollate broth and are labeled aerobic (oxygen present) and anarobic (no oxygen present). The vial labeled aerobic checks for bacteria which requires oxygen o survive.

anarobic. The vial labeled aerobic checks for bacteria which requires oxygen to survive. The vial labeled anarobic checks for oraganisms which cannot survive when oxygen is present. Upon collection the vials are then placed into an incubator for twenty four hours. The microbiologist will view each for for the presence of bacteria and will report their findings to the ordering physician. Other common tests performed are.

Culture and Sensitivity (C&S): The primary function of a urine culture and sensitivity test is to aid in detecting urinary tract infections as well as bladder infections. Specimens must be collected in a sterile cup using a clean catch mid-stream collection to prevent the possibility of a false positive.

Throat Culture: The purpose of a throat culture is to detect streptococcal (strep) infections. Throat cultures are collected in a kit which contains a polyester tipped swab. Upon swabbing the back of the throat the swab is then placed back into the transport tube and sent to the lab for testing. When doctors need results quickly a rapid strep test is performed at the facility. Results of a rapid strep test are within five minutes.

Ova and Parasite: When a patent exhibits persistant diarrhea or other intestinal symptoms, the healthcare provider may order an ova and parasite test. The stool is collected in a plastic bowl an then transferred into specimen containers. Upon receipt of the specimen, the lab will take a sample and place it under a microscope to see if any parasites are present.

Coagulation Lab: The coagulation lab studies the bodies ability to clot as well as monitor blood thinners such as Coumadin or Heparin The following are some of the most common tests performed. Be mindful that a light blue top tube is collected for coagulation studies. These tubes must be full (**no exceptions**). Light blue tubes are inverted six to eight times to mix the anticoagulant with the blood.

Prothrombin Time (PT): Prothrombin time is a the screening of choice for monitoring anticoagulant therapy.

Abnormal results may indicate, hepatic disease, deficiencies in vitamin K, fibrinogen, prothrombin.

Platelet count: Platelets aid in blood clotting. Low platelet counts can be due to leukemia, vitamin K deficiency, celiac disease or chemotherapy. An increase of platelets may be due to anemia, primary thrombocythemia (the production of too many platelets in the bone marrow).

Activated Partial Thromboplastin Time (APTT): An APTT is a test used to monitor heparin therapy. Abnormal results may be due to the presence of heparin a deficiency in certain plasma clotting clotting factors.

Now that you have been introduced to the various departments in a laboratory and some of their functions, let's now begin exploring some of the complications and other factors to consider prior to and during, a blood collection.

Chapter 3

Factors and complications to consider prior to a venipuncture

In this chapter we will discuss some of the factors and possible complications you need to be aware of before performing a venipuncture. You will also learn some important techniques to manage some of the complications you may encounter during a venipuncture.

Age: Age sometimes can be a challenge. As a person ages they may lose muscle tone as in geriatric patients. Their veins may roll away from the puncture site causing the needle to miss the vein. The best way to handle a roll away vein is simply by pulling the skin downwards, this will cause the vein to straighten out allowing you to insert the needle into the vein with ease. A word of caution, should you miss the vein you should avoid moving the needle around as this can cause a hematoma (bruise) as well as further trauma. If you were unsuccessful in obtaining blood, remove the needle, hold pressure for ten seconds and try another site or ask for help from a more experienced phlebotomist.

Pediatric patients can be challenging as well, simply for the fact that depending on the child's age phlebotomy can be a challenge. For instance some pediatric veins can be small which can make can make bloodletting a challenge however, what can make bloodletting more challenging is the fact that the needle be very frightening to the child. Unlike an adult who understands the purpose of phlebotomy children think differently, in their mind you are about to insert an object they not familiar with therefore you need to be empathetic and understand what they are thinking which is "Why are you doing this to me?" Therefore there should always be a second phlebotomist when attempting to draw blood from a child, one to hold the child's arm and the other to perform the venipuncture.

Dehydration: Dehydration can occur when a patient lacks fluid intake or is vomiting or has severe diarrhea. Dehydration can make bloodletting difficult because many times the vein can collapse upon insertion of the needle. The best way to remdy this situation is ask the patient to intake some fluids and reattempt bloodletting fifteen minutes after fluid intake. Many times fluid intake resolve the problem.

Scars, Burns and Tattooed areas: Try to avoid areas, with scars, burns or tattoos especially if the scar, burn, or tattoo is fresh because the possibility of infection is high.

Mastectomy (Breast removal): Avoid blood from an arm where a mastectomy has been performed. This is because lymph nodes have been removed from the site where the mastectomy has been performed. This can cause the patient to develop an infection. Many times the patient will tell you if they had a mastectomy. In this case simply look for a vein on the opposite arm. For patients who have had a double mastectomy, avoid the side where the mastectomy was recently performed.

Obesity: phlebotomy on an obese patient can be a challenge because the veins may be deep, sometimes a warm cloth or warm compress will aid in locating a vein. Another remedy is have the patient rotate their arm so that the hand is facing prone this may in some cases help the excess tissue and weight fall downward making it easier to locate the cephalic vein.

Damaged veins: Damaged veins can be caused by many factors such as chronic illness or over use of a vein. Damaged veins may have no bounce too them or they may feel like a cord. In this cirmunstance locate a vein below the damaged area or try the opposite arm.

Edema (swelling): Edema is caused by fluid buildup in the tissues. Edema can be associated with several factors such as heart failure (HF). Heart failure is when the heart does not maintain adequate blood flow. Some medications such as hormone replacements, nonsteroidal anti-inflammatory drugs (NSAIDS) can cause edema. Other factors such as a high salt intake or immobility can also cause edema.

Hematoma (Bruise): A hematoma is a mass of blood caused by blood leaking from a blood vessel. If possible, avoid bloodletting from a site with a hematoma. A hematoma can be caused by extensive use of vein such as hospitalization where bloodletting is often performed or improper insertion of the needle (going through the vein or overpuncturing the vein with the same needle) this is when the needle is shifted in many directions. Should you encounter a site with a hematoma search for a vein on the opposite arm. If you have no other alternative but to use the arm with a hematoma try going distal (below) the hematoma this will help minimize pain and further trauma to the site.

Intravenous line (IV): At some point throughout your career you may encounter a patient with an intravenous line. In this situation alway's, ask the nurse in charge if you have permission to draw blood. One reason is because the vein accessed may be the only good vein, therefore, the nurse will draw blood from the line. In most cases however, you will be permitted to draw blood on the opposite arm or below the IV line. Prior to the venipuncture, ask the nurse to shut down the line for about two minutes and collect a discard tube this is because the blood may become diluted from the fluids which can result in inaccurate test results.

Possible complications:

Although most of the time you will perform a complete venipuncture procedure without incident I can assure you will encounter complications from time to time. Nonetheless, you must always be prepared to act upon any complications swiftly. Let's begin exploring some of the most common complications in detail.

Syncope (Fainting/vasovagal response): Syncope is a result in the sudden decline in blood pressure and it is without any doubt that during your career as a phlebotomist that you will encounter a patient who develops syncope. Let's now explore some of the reasons why a patient may faint otherwise known as syncope or vasovagal response along with some tips which may help prevent syncope.

Dehydration: Inadequate hydration can cause the patient to become dizzy or lightheaded or faint as bloodletting begins. this is due to a decrease in the level of body fluids along with a decline in blood pressure as well as the of some blood causing insufficient blood flow to the brain causing a temporary vasovagal response.

Anxiety: Anxiety associated with phlebotomy is usually due to fear, such as seeing the sight of their own blood or just observing the needle can cause to patient to become tense and ultimately develop syncope. Many patients have had a prior negative experience.

Diet: low blood sugar such as diabetes or fasting prior to a venipuncture can cause a sudden drop in blood pressure causing the patient to experience syncope.

To prevent syncope here are some tips to follow.

- Speak to the patient during before, during, and after a venipuncture. Speaking to the patient will help keep the patient's mind off of the procedure, minimizing anxiety and possibly possibly preventing syncope.

- Should the patient feel light headed or dizzy ask the patient to remain seated, and to lean forward, and place their head between their knees. This position will help to increase blood circulation to the brain resulting in reduced risk of syncope.

Should syncopy occur, stop the procedure immediately, call for help. Never under any circumstance leave the patient unattended until medical help arrives. For detailed procedures go to www.fundementals of phlebotomy.com and click on phlebotomy procedures. Then click on link for syncope.

Hematoma: A hematoma is caused by blood leaking in the tissues around the venipuncture site causing a bruise to occur. A hematoma can cause damage to the nerves and can be painful and can be caused by the following.

- Inserting the needle through the vein
- Excessive probing
- Blind probing
- The needle is inserted partly into the vein
- Not applying pressure following the venipuncture
- Not removing the tourniquet before the needle

Excessive bleeding: Most often patients will stop bleeding shortly after a venipuncture. However, patients on asprin therapy or blood thinners such as Coumadin may take longer to stop bleeding. Therefore, prior to drawing blood ask the patient if he/she is on any blood thinners including aspirin. Upon completion apply extra gauze on the site and ask the patient to apply direct pressure. It is recommended that the patient remain in the waiting area for five minutes and observe the puncture site prior to the patient leaving. If the bleeding continues notify a nurse or other healthecare provider about the situation.

Seizures: Although rare, you may encounter a patient having a seizure during a venipuncture However, in the event a seizure should occur, immediately remove the needle and call for assistance. Following the seizure the patient should be examined by a healthecare provider to ensure proper patient management.

Nausea/Vomiting: In some rare cases a patient may complain of nausea during or after bloodletting. In this case try and talk with the patient and hand them an emesis basin. Should the patient vomit call for immediate medical assistance and monitor the patients blood pressure.

Infection: Although rare, an infection can occur at the venipuncture site. Therefore, to minimize the possibility of an infection occuring, properly clean the site prior to the venipuncture and immediately place gauze on the puncture site after. To prevent bacteria from entering the site ask the patient to keep the gauze on for ten to fifteen minutes, twenty minutes or longer for patient's on blood thinners. If the patient refuses bandage on the site explain to them it is for their safety and that they can remove the bandage shortly after leaving the facility.

Remember, the venipuncture procedure is not complete until the bandage is placed on the site.

Collapsed Vein: Several factors can cause a collapsed vein to occur. For example, placing the tourniquet to close to the venipuncture site or when a patient is dehydrated. Elderly patients are another group where a collapsed vein can occur, this is because the veins are fragile and they loose their elasticity. Sometimes the pressure of the vacutainer tube can cause a vein to colllapse. Where permissable, a pediatric tube can be used especially for veins that cannot withstand the pressure of full size vacutainer.

Now that we have covered some of the most common factors and complications that may arise during a venipuncture procedure, let us now explore some of the factors which may affect the basal state (factors which affect the components of the blood).

Smoking: Smoking can increase the level of hemoglobin due to carbon monoxide (a by-product of tobacco smoke). In some cases due to poor circulation, obtaining a blood sample from a finger may be difficult especialy from chronic smokers.

Stress: Patients who exhibit stress due to anxiety can cause a decrease in the number of white blood cells (leukocytes). Therefore try to keep the patient calm is important, such as talking with the patient, talking to the patient helps by keeping their mind off of the procedure.

Medications: Several medications can alter the physiological function of the blood components. For example, chemotherapy medications decrease white blood and platelet counts, where other medications can cause potassium levels to drop, for this reason it is common for a provider to monitor the levels of blood components while a patient is receiving chemotherapy.

Diet: The diet a person is on greatly affects the results of many laboratory tests. For example, when a person eats foods with a fatty substance such as butter, this can cause the plasma or serum to appear cloudy (lipemic) due to the increase of lipids in the blood. Therefore, the accuracy of the test may be diminished.

Some tests require that the specimen be collected at a specific time while other tests will take priority. Let's explore the following designations.

STAT: The term STAT means that the specimen should be drawn and tested immediately. For example, if a patients conditio changes from serious to critical condition the physician may order a Coumadin level and needs the results STAT. Therefore, the lab test will be performed STAT usually within an hour and reported to the patient caregiver.

ASAP (as soon as possible): Specimens which are not considered STAT but are considered serious may be ordered ASAP. ASAP lab tests are usually completed within two hours.

Routine: Routine labs are generally performed during a physical examination or to monitoring the patient's medication. Therefore, the test results are not immediatly needed. Routine tests are usually completed within twenty-four to forty-eight hours.

Pre-op/ Post-op: Pre-op and post-op labs are performed to detect if there are any infections present prior to surgery and after surgery as well as checking the patients overall general state of health. The following basic post-op and pre-op tests are usually performed. Additionally, depending on the type of surgery, other specific lab tests may be performed for example, following liver surgery, a liver function test may be ordered.

Complete cloood count (CBC):

A CBC is performed to detect anemia, dehydration or infections. A CBC includes the following tests.

Red blood cell count (RBC): Red blood cells carry oxygen to the body. Low RBC count can indicate, leukemia, malnutrition or problems with the bone marrow. A high RBC count can indicate, kidney disease, dehydration, heart problems or over transfusion.

White blood cell count (WBC): White blood cells help fight infection and also play a role in inflammation. A low WBC count can indicate, autoimmune disease, problems with the liver or spleen, autoimmune disease or chemical exposure. A high WBC count can indicate, leukemia, infectious disease or tissue damage.

Hematocrit (HCT): Hematocrits are the percentage of blood that is composed of red blood cells. Low hematocrits can indicate anemia, blood loss, bone marrow problems, malnutrition. A high hematocrit count can indicate dehydration, living in high altitudes, congenital heart disease, smoking, polycythemia (overproduction of red blood cells).

Hemoglobin (Hgb): Hemoglobn is a protein in the red blood cells that carry oxygen. Low levels of hemoglobin can indicate blood loss or anemia.

Platelets (PLT) (thrombocytes): Platelets are a part of the blood that make the blood clot. Low platelets can indicate leukemia, chemotherapy, recent transfusion. High levels can indicate certain types of cancer, polycythemia, anemia.

Sedimentation Rate (Sed rate): Sedimentation rate also known as an Erythrocyte Sedimentation Rate (ESR) measures how quickly red blood cells fall to the bottom of a test tube. Physicians use this test to detect and monior inflammation of the body. A Sedimentation rate is also used to monitor the treatment and progress of a disease such a rheumatoid arthritis.

Fasting: From time to time healthcare providers may order tests which require a patient to not consume food or drinks (with the exception of water or medications). This would also include no smoking or chewing gum between eight to twelve hours prior to the test. Therefore, most fasting lab tests are performed in the morning, this is so the patient does not go wothout food for a long period of time. Never under any circumstance should you advise a patient to stop taking their medications, the healthcare provider will instruct the patient to continue or discontinue taking their medication. Some common fasting lab tests are glucose, lipid levels such as cholesterol, tirglycerides, and HDL.

Chapter 4

Infection Control and Safety

In this chapter we will discuss in depth about healthcare safety and first aid including preventing infection commonly known as infection control. Let's begin with laboratory safety rules.

In 1970 the Occupational Safety and Health Administration (OSHA) mandated that all healthcare employers set up safe working conditions for their employees.

Therefore, following all precautions and safety rules will aid in the prevention of injuries to you as well as the patient.

Laboratory safety rules:

- Handle all specimens with standard safety precautions (treat all specimens as infectious).
- Always wear gloves during specimen collection or specimen transfer.
- Never consume any food or drink In the laboratory.
- Never apply contact lens or cosmetics in the laboratory. (cross contamination can occur).
- Always wear a lab coat (fully buttoned) and never wear a lab coat outside of the laboratory.

- Wear a face shield, lab coat, and gloves when working with specimens that might splash.
- Hair over shoulder length must be tied back.
- Avoid wearing long dangling or large earrings, long chains, loose bracelets.
- No food or beverages in a refrigerator or freezer designated for storing specimens.
- Nail polish or artificial nails should never be worn, especially in phlebotomy. Nails should be kept short, and never bite nails.
- Wear shoes that are comfortable and nonslip. Never wear high heals, sandals or shoes with open toes.

Safety rules when entering a patients room:

- All specimens must be handled with standard safety precautions.
- Always wear gloves when collecting specimens or when handling bedding.
- Bedrails must always be placed in the upright position after completion of any procedure.
- Report unresponsive patients to nursing.
- Properly dispose of all contaminated supplies in the proper containers (ie, needles in sharps containers, soiled gauze in biohazard bag, in patient's rooms).
- Report any spills to nursing and housekeeping.
- Report odors to nursing and if necessary to houskeeping.
- Wear protective gear when prompted to (ie face mask, gown).
- Never eat patients food even when offered.

Infection Control

Infection: The enviroment we live in is full of microscopic organisms called microbes. Microbes include fungi, bacteria, protozoa, and viruses. A disease causing microbe is called pathogenic meaning the microbe has the capability of causing disease. An infection that acts on the body is called a local infection. An infection that affects the entire body is called a systemic infection.

Nosocomial Infections: Nosocomial infections occur inside hospitals or healthcare facilities and result when patients healthcare providers and personnel, including visitors come in contact with an infected person. Therefore, safety precautions recommended by the Centers for Disease Control and prevention (CDC) should be adhered to.

Chain of infection: An infection occurs when the following components known as a chain of infection are present. In order for an infection to occur, all the components must exist. Let's explore each component in detail.

Etiologic agent: Agents that can cause infectious diseases, etiological agents, are also referred to as causative agents. There are several types of agents which are capable of causing infectious diseases. They are; bacteria, fungi, viruses, metazoa, protozoa, and rickettsia. Etiological agents are also known as the source of infection.

- **Bacteria:** Bacteria is a single-celled organism with nucleus and is capable of causing a wide range of human disease such as tuberculosis, staphyloccocal disease, tetanus, diptheria, chlamydia, and many more.

- **Fungi:** Fungi are organisms which can cause diseases and can be very difficult to treat. For example, candidiasis which is a fungus which causes lesions on the skin or mucous membranes such as thrush.

- **Viruses:** Viruses are very small and can only reproduce and grow inside of living cells. Viruses include: influenza, measels, mumps, rubella, rabies, and HIV.

- **Metazoa:** Metazoa's are multicullar animals of which many are parasites such as hookworm and trichinellosis.

- **Protozoa:** Protozoa's ar a single-celled organism with a nucleus. Some diseases caused by protozoa's are; pneumonia, malaria, giardiasis (an infection of the upper small intestine).

- **Rickettsia:** Rickettsia is a bacteria found in the cells of lice, ticks, mites, and fleas.

Reservoir: A reservoir is the source where an infectious agent lives and multiplies. Reservoirs may be human, animals, or enviromental. Let's begin with human reservoirs.

Human: Human reservoirs can be acute cases or carrier. Acute cases are humans who may be infected with an agent and become ill and in most cases will be diagnosed and treated.

Carriers: There are five types of carriers; Incubatory carrier, inapparent infections, convalescent carriers, and chronic carriers. Let's explore each one in detail.

Incubatory carrier: Incubatory carriers can begin transmitting an infection even before symptoms begin to appear. For example, a person infected with HIV can transmit the disease even before symptoms appear.

Inapparent infections: When people contract inapparent infections they may never develop symptoms however, the disease can still be tramsmitted to others. For example, hepatitis A which is passed through feces even without symptoms.

Convalescent carriers: People who are convalescent carriers may continue to be infectious even after the illness has passed such as salmonella which can be passed through feces weeks after recovery.

Chronic carriers: People who continue to be infectious for more than a year are chronic carriers such as hepatitis B which can be tranmitted by blood products, sexually, infected needles, toiletries (such as a toothbrush).

Animal reservoirs: Like humans, animal reservoirs of infectious agents can be transmitted to humans. In fact there are over one hundred pathogenic species of bacteria that can both humans and animals and like humans animals can be both acute or carriers depanding on the disease. For example, rabies animals can spread the virus three to five days prior to developing symptoms.

Enviromental: Soil, plants, and water can also serve as a reservoir of infection. For example tetanus, a common bacteria found in the soil which if not treated can cause nerve aliments.

Mode of transmission: Mode of transmission is the means in which the infectious agent escapes. They are, contact transmission, airborne transmission, droplet transmission, vehicle transmission, and vector transmission.

Contact transmission: Contact transmission is the most common mode of infection transmission and there are two types of transmissions, direct and indirect transmission.

Direct transmission: Direct transmission is when a pathogenic microbe is transferred physically to a susceptible host. For example, touching (ie; kissing or shaking hands). It should be noted that direct transmission is the most common form if transmission.

Indirect transmission: Indirect transmission is when the susceptible host has contact with an inanimate object which may be infected with infectious microbes. such as eating utensils, door knob, bed linen, and needles, just to name a few.

Droplet transmission: Droplet transmission is the transfer of an infectious microbe to a susceptible host through the mucous membranes of the mouth, nose or the conjunctiva (mucous membrane of the eye). Transmission occurs through sneezing, coughing or talking.

Airborne transmission: Airborne transmission is the spreading of droplet nuclei, this occurs through sneezing, talking, and coughing. Unlike droplet transmission the droplets only travel a few feet where as with airborne transmission the microbes become widely spread before being inhaled by the susceptible host. It is also important to note that the droplet nuclei are capable of remaining suspended in the air for a long period of time, therefore, a proper fitted mask with a special filter must be worn before entering a patient's room. Some examples of airborne transmission droplets are, varicella (chicken pox), and tuberculosis.

Vector transmission: Vector transmission is when infectious microbes are transmitted by an Insect or animal for example, an infected mosquito can transmit the West Nile virus or malaria.

Vehicle transmission: Vehicle transmission involves contaminated water, food, or drugs for example, typhoid fever, shigella, and cholera can be transmitted by drinking comtaminated water. You should also note that receiving contaminated blood products is also considered vehicle transmission.

Susceptible host: Depending on the age, health and immune status of a patient determines how susceptible a person may be. For example, the elderly may have an immune system which is no longer functioning properly or newborns, their immune system is not fully developed, therefore, they are more susceptible to infections where as a healthy person who is updated with their vaccinations or has recovered from a virus, has developed antibodies against that particular virus, in this case the person is said to be immune.

The chain of infection can be broken by beginning at the source. This is accomplished by proper handwashing, wearing gloves, gown, face shield and other personel protective equipment (PPE), proper decontamination of equipment and surfaces, and proper waste disposal will greatly reduce risk of infection.

Occupational exposure of infection to the health care worker is a serious matter, therefore, to prevent health risks, you must follow standard precautions when working in any healthcare setting. Occuupational Safety and Health Administration (OSHA) has concluded that exposure to occupational blood and blood products in the health care setting is high. Therefore, OSHA has put into force a bloodborne pathogen standard and is mandated by federal law. The purpose of the standard is to help minimize as well as eliminate the to viruses such as hepatitis B and AIDS. Another organization JCAHO (the Joint Commission on the accreditation of health organizations) sets and implements procedures to every health care organization. These procedures are designed to protect the heath care workers, patients, and visitors. Let's now explore the bloodborne pathogens, transmission of bloodborne pathogens, and standard precautions.

Parenteral Transmission: Parenteral transmission is the means or route a bloodborne pathogenic enters. They are as follows: Percutanious (through the skin), nonintact skin, and mucous membrane. Parenteral transmission however, does not include the digestive tract however, does include human bites which penetrate the skin therefore, injecting blood which can be potentially infectious.

Percutanious: Percutanious is the direct transmission of blood or blood products through broken tubes containing blood as well as accidental needle sticks.

Nonintact skin: Infectious pathogen can also enter the skin through visible as well as invisible cracks and cuts on the skin, such as chapped lips and hands, scratches and burns. It's for this reason gloves must be worn to prevent the posibility of contracting an infection.

Mucous membrane: This is when the mucosa of the nose, mouth and conjunctiva eyes become introduced with an infectious agent either by droplets, splashes, touching of the mouth, nose, and eyes can also introduce an infectious agent.

Bloodborne Pathogens: As previously mentioned, being a healthcare worker you may be exposed to body fluids especially in the laboratory. Let's explore the most common pathogens a healthcare worker can be exposed to.

Human Immunodeficiency Virus (HIV): HIV is capable of disabeling the immune system and is the primary cause of AIDS (Aquired Immuno Deficiency Syndrome).

Hepatitis B virus (HBV): HBV is the most common infection associated with the laboratory. HBV attacks the liver and can be potentially fatal. In fact the HBV virus can survive for up to one week even in dry blood. Therefore, it is highly recommended that the healthcare worker be vaccinated for hepatitis B. In fact OSHA requires that all heathcare institutions offer the employee the hepatitis B vaccine at no cost.

Tuberculosis (TB): Tuberculosis is caused by the myobacterium (*tuberculosis bacterium*) and is spread through the air from person to person. Although TB is contagious but is difficult to catch. As a healthcare worker you must always protect yourself. Following the directios of the nursing staff as well as any signs posted. You must also wear a special protective mask to prevent exposure.

OSHA Laboratory Standards: As previously mentioned, Occupational Safety and Health Administration (OSHA) has put into force the occupational exposure to bloodborne pathogens standard and is mandated by federal law. The stanndard is to help minnimize occupational hazards such as wearing personal protective equipment (PPE) (eg; lab coat to protect clothing or face shield to protect the face from potential splashing of body fluids). Confidential medical evaluation, treatment and counseling has halso been mandated by OSHA. This now takes us to infection control.

Handwashing: Understanding when hands should be washed will aid in the prevention and the spread of infection, therefore hands should be washed:

- Before and after a procedure or contact with a patient. This also includes when performing multiple procedures on the same patient (eg; urinalysis followed by a venipuncture).
- Before putting on and after taking off gloves.
- Before and after going to the restroom.
- Before and after lunch or break.
- Before leaving the laboratory.
- When hands have been contaminated.

Proper handwashing technique: The following routine handwashing technique should never be altered, **NO EXCEPTIONS.**

- Remove jewelryy (including watch).
- Wet hands under running, warm water.
- Apply soap and lather (Sing Happy Birthday). 20 seconds
- Rub hands to create friction, this will help loosen any dirt or dead skin.
- Scrub everywhere, for 20 seconds this includes between the fingers as well as around the knuckles.
- Rinse hands, allowing the soap to run down. Do not re-touch hands as this could cause recontamination.
- Dry hands with a clean paper towel.
- Turn faucet off using with a clean paper towel.

Protective gear:

Here we will discuss some of the gear known as personal protective equipment (PPE). Some of the gear is as needed and some are required by OSHA.

Gloves: Gloves are an essential PPE when performing phlebotomy or handling any body fluids. Generally the gloves are nonsterile and latex free. Gloves are worn to protect the hands from possible contamination. The gloves should feel comfortable and cover the entire hand. Under no circumstance should you tear the index finger portion of the glove. This method can cause recontamination to the site as well as causing the finger to be exposed to body fluids. Afterwords, the gloves should be removed by grasping the wrist portion of the glove, turning the glove inside out. With the other hand put one finger under the wrist portion of the glove and remove the glove inside out. The gloves should then be disposed of properly.

Mask: A mask is worn to protect the nose and mouth from droplets caused by coughing or sneezing. The mask must be secure and able to cover the nose and mouth.

Respirator: From time to time you may be called to enter a room where a patient may have tuberculosis or other type of airborn disease. Therefore, before entering the room you must wear a properly fitted N95 respirator. The respirator provides a snug fit preventing air leaks from occuring.

Goggles/faceshields: Goggles are worn to protect the eyes from possible splashes or sprays of body fluids. Faceshields are worn to portect the eyes mouth and nose from possibe sprays and splashes of body fluids. Although, goggles and faceshields are not mandatory they should be worn whenever splashing or spraying can occur, such as performing urinalysis.

Lab coat/gown: Lab coats must always be clean and are worn to protect personal clothing from possible contamination from splashes and sprays. Under no circumstance should a lab coat be worn outside of the lab, doing so can cause possible contamination of a clean area. Gowns are generallly nonsterile fluid resistant and are worn to prevent contamination of personal clothing. Some healthcare workers are required to wear sterile gowns to protect patients with a weak immune system, such as infants.

Chapter 5

The Blood Drawing Station

In this chapter we will discuss a typical blod drawing station, the supplies needed, as well as the various bloood collection tubes, the additives and their function along with the proper amount of inversions before samples are sent off for technical analysis.

Blood collection stations vary, for example, blood collection stations in an academic hospital or health facility may have more blood drawing stations because of the volume of patients. Whereas, in a small private office the blood drawing station may only need one phlebotomist. Nonetheless, the station includes a phlebotomy chair as welll as a reclining chaiir for patients with a history of syncope (fainting). Typically, each blood drawing station carries the following supplies. Let's discuss the equipment required for a venipuncture procedure.

Gloves: The Occupational Safety and Health Administration (OSHA), along with the Centers for Disease Control and Prevention, require that all persons handling blood and and body fluids must wear gloves. The gloves should feel comfortable as well as fit the contour of your hand, for example large gloves will have a loose fitting on a medium size hand whereas small gloves will be too tight. Another reason for proper fitted gloves is gloves larger than the hand can get in the way of the blood procedure especially when performing a capillary puncture (fingerstick).

Antiseptics: Antiseptic solutions are used to prevent sepsis (infection) and are used prior to a venipuncture or capillary puncture. The following antiseptics are used:

- **70% Isopropyl alcohol (isopropanol):** This is the most common antiseptic used and are contained in individual wrappers. It should be noted that if a patient is being tested for blood alcohol levels, isopropyl alcohol should not be used as it can cause a false positive for alcohol therefore, povidone-iodine should be used.

- **Povidone-iodine:** povidone-iodine comes in sponge pads or swab sticks and are used when performing a blood culture, blood gas collection or when isopropyl alcohol should not be used such as blood alcohol levels.

- Gauze pads: 2 X 2 gauze pads are used after the venipuncture is complete. The pad is folded into fourths. The gauze will cover the puncture site as well as prevent bleeding. You should always ask the patient if he/she is on any blood thinners or asprin therapy as they can case the site to continue bleeding longer. Should you experience a patient on blood blood thinners or asprin therapy, simply place extra gauze on the site. The patient should keep the gauze on for 10-15 minutes and 20-30 minutes for patients on thinners or asprin.

- **Bandage:** Bandages are used to to keep the gauze in place or directly over the puncture puncture site. Types of bandage used are paper or cloth. Most often paper tape is used because it has a small amount of adhesive and is less traumatic to the skin. Another type of bandage is coban this gauze sticks to itself and not the skin.

  Coban is typically used when performing an arterial bloood gas or after an infusion such as chemotherapy, however, coban can be used after a venipuncture. A word of caution, bandages should not be used on childern younger than 2 years of age due to the risk of aspiration.

- **Sharps containers:** All sharps or biohazard containers should be pre-approved by OSHA. The red sharps containers are puncture and leak proof and marked "Biohazard". There are different styles of sharps containers, some are wall mounted while some are floor models. They also have a "fill line", therefore, sharps should never go beyond the fill line to prevent an accidental needle stick. Sharps are supposed be dropped in the biohazard container - not shoved into the container.

- **Tourniquet:** The purpose of a tourniquet is when applied will cause the vein to enlarge, allowing you to palpate (feel) the vein and allow easy insertion of the needle into the vein. Tourniquets come in adult and pediatric size and it should be noted that the tourniquet should never be left on for more than one minute to prevent hemolysis (destruction of red blood cells). Should a tourniquet be unavailable, a blood pressure cuff can be used, simply by applying 15-20 mm/hg of pressure.

- **Needles:** Phlebotomy needles include multisample needles and winged infusion (butterfly needles). Multisample needles should always be used before using winged infusion needles because the lumen of a butterfly needle is smaller and can cause hemolysis (Destruction of red blood cells). Lets now explore the parts of a needle.

- **The gauge:** The gauge of the needle determines the size of the needle and also refers to the diameter of the lumen or bore (internal space of the needle). The gauge of the needle determines the actual diameter of the needle. The larger the number the smaller the diameter of the needle. For example a

22g needle is smaller than a 21g needle. The typical gauge used is 21g and 22g.

- **The bevel:** The bevel of the needle is cut at a slant to allow easy penetration of the needle through the skin and into the vein. The bevel also prevents coring (removal of a portion of skin or vein).

- **The shaft/hub:** The shaft is the long cylinder portion of the needle and is connected to the hub the apparatus which draws the blood.

Now that we have reviewed the parts of the needle let's review the components of an evacuated test tube system.

A complete evacuated test tube system includes a multisample needle, a tube holder, and the evacuated test tube.

The evacuated test tube system consists of a beveled point on both ends of a needle with a threaded middle. The threaded portion of the needle allows easy attachment to the holder referred to as the adaptor. One end of the needle will penetrate the skin where the other end which has a retractable rubbed sleeve will penetrate the test tube. The sleeve also prevents blood from leaking out of the adaptor when changing test tubes. All needles are sterile, sealed, and color coded along with gauge identification. The needles come in two sizes, 1 inch and 1 ½ inches. The gauges most often used in phlebotomy are 21g and 22g. Determining the size, and gauge of the needle depends on the size of the vein, this is predetermined by palpating (feeling the vein).

The clear plastic cylinder known as the test tube holder or adapter has a small opening to thread the needle, the wider opening is for the tube. The test tube holder is available in standard size and pediatric size. The holders are one time use and should never be used between patients due to possible contamination.

The test tube fills with blood due to a vacuum inside the tube. The vacuum is premeasured and is guaranteed by the manufacturer until the expiration date printed on the tube. Most tubes are made of plastic to prevent breakage and range from 2ml to 15ml. To determine the proper size tube to use determines the age of the patient and condition of the vein, (ie; use small tubes for pediatric veins).

Collection tubes and order of draw: Here we will discuss the additives some of the tubes contain, the purpose of the additive, and the proper order of draw. It is imperative that you understand the proper order of draw. Incorrect order of draw could cause contamination of an additive from one tube to another ultimately affecting the test results. Let's now begin exploring in detail the tube additives, their purpose and proper order of draw. For valuable information go to Quest Diagnostics.com and click on order of draw. You can also go to

Blood Culture tubes: When ordered, blood cultures are always drawn first. The specimens are collected in bottles which contain a soybean casin broth with CO_2 which promotes growth of any organism present in the blood. Generally blood cultures are collect in sets of two. The bottles are marked anaerobic (organisms that require no oxygen to survive) and aerobic (organisms that require oxygen to survive). The preparation of the blood draw site requires a sterile technique by using povidone-iodine. When cleaning the site, always begin from the center, mover the debris outward using a spiral motion. Under no circumstances should the area be touched as this will recontaminate the site. If repalpating the site is necessary, sterile gloves must be worn. As the area is drying begin cleaning the tops of the bottles with povidone-iodine and place a clean alcohol wipe on the bottle until ready to use. When ready to draw blood, use a clean alcohol wipe to clean the tops of the bottles, this is so the iodine is not introduced into the blood culture bottle. For pediatric patients, only one bottle is collected however the preparation is the same.

Serum Separator Tube (SST)/Plasma Separator Tube (PST): The Serum Separator Tube contains a thixotropic gel (a nonreacting substance that when activated, creates a barrier between the cellular and serum or plasma components of the specimen). When properly centrifuged, the gel forms a barrier between the serum or plasma. Gel tubes which separate serum have a red/gray top also known a mottled, some also refer this tube as a tiger top tube because of the red/gray stripes on the stopper. Gel tubes which separate plasma known as a Plasma Separator Tube (PST) have a gray/green stopper. SST/PST test tubes should be inverted five times gently.

Lavender top tube: Lavender top tubes contain the anticoagulant (prevents clotting) Ethylenediaminetetraacetic acid (EDTA). EDTA prevents clotting by binding calcium in the form of potassium or sodium salt. EDTA also preserves cell morphology and prevents platlets from clumping together. Lavender top tubes should be gently inverted eight to ten times for proper mixing of agent with blood.

Light blue tubes: Light blue top tubes contain Sodium Citrate. Sodium Citrate binds with calcium to prevent coagulation (clotting) and is used for coagulation studies (ie; coumadin level). Before drawing a light blue top tube, a discard tube should be drawn to prevent possible dilution of the sample but, most importantly, the light blue top tube MUST always be completly fill **No Exceptions**. The lab will not perform the test if the tube is received partly filled. This will cause the test to be delayed and a need for a redraw. The light blue top tubes should be gently inverted inverted three to four times for proper mixing of agent with blood.

Green top tubes: Green top tubes and royal blue top tubes with a green band contain heparin. Heparin prevents clotting (coagulation) by not allowing prothrombin to convert to thrombin. There are three formulations of heparin, lithium, ammonia, and sodium. Green top tubes should be inverted eight to ten times gently for proper mixing of agent with blood.

Gray top tubes: Gray top tubes contain ammonium oxalate or potassium which prevent clotting by separating calcium. Gray top tubes are generally used for glucose testing. Gray top tubes should be inverted eight to ten times gently for proper mixing of agent with blood.

Order of Draw: To reduce the possibility of additive crossover between tubes, the order of draw was established. The crossover of additives occurs when a tube containing an additive comes in contact with the stopper puncture needle, therefore, transferring additives between tubes. The most common addditive contamination is EDTA. EDTA can cause a false increase in coagulation levels, this is also true with heparin contamination. Therefore, remembering the order of draw is vital. After collecting blood, remember that proper tube inversion is equally important as the order of draw. Proper order of draw and tube inversion proceeds as follows.

Blood culture bottles (sterile)
Light blue (sodium citrate) Tube must be fill Invert 3-4 times gently
Serum Separator Tube (SST) Invert 5 times gently
Red (contains no additive
Green (heparin) Invert 8-10 times gently
Lavender (EDTA) Invert 8-10 times gently
Royal Blue (EDTA) Invert 8-10 times gently
Gray (sodium fluoride) Invert 8-10 times gently
Yellow (citrate ACD) Invert 3-4 times gently.

Order of draw can also be previewed by going to Quest diagnostics order of draw. You will not only find the proper order of draw, you can also obtain a wealth of information regarding various tests and proper collection tubes as well as proper tube handling. You can also view proper order of draw by going to www.phlebotomyfundamentalscom and click on order of draw.

Chapter 6

Phlebotomy

In this chapter we will discuss the most commonly veins used in phlebotomy as well as other possible locations phlebotomy can be performed. We will also discuss in detail the fourteen steps to a complete phlebotomy procedure. Remember, phlebotomy is an art and a science and must be practiced until mastered. Therefore, in this chapter, pay close attention to the details and put them into action with precision. Let's begin.

Antecubital Fossa (bend of the arm): The veins most commonly used in phlebotomy are located in the antecubital fossa. The veins are the Median cubital vein, cephalic vein, and basilic vein. Let's cover each vein in detail.

Median cubital vein: The median cubital vein also referred to as the cubital vein is located in the center of the elbow and is a connection for th cephalic vein and basislic vein. The median cubital vein is the preferred vein in phlebotomy because the site is less painful and the chance of vein rollover is less likley to occur. The median cubital vein should be your first choice vein.

Cephalic vein: The vein of second choice is the cephalic vein it runs from the lateral (side) of the arm from the hand to the shoulder. Like the median cubital vein, the cephalic vein is less painfull, however, anchoring (hold in place) the ven is recommended for easy insertion of the needle.

Basilic vein: The third choice of veins is the basilic vein. The basilic vein runs from the shoulder and elbow and is located on the same side as the brachial artery. The site is more painfull and the possibility of a hematoma (bruise) is more likely to occur. Because the vein is close to the bracial artery extra caution should be observed. Should an accidental puncture of an artery occur quickly remove the needle and apply pressure. Here is a tip, if the vessel is pulsating, then it is not a vein, it is an artery.

Other phlebotomy sites: When the veins of the antecubital fossa are not accessable, veins of the arms, hands, and sometimes the wrist can be used. Let's explore these sites.

Arm: When searching for a vein in the arm, check both the anterior (front) and posterior (back) of the arm for a suitable vein. Upon locating a vein begin preperation for blood drawing. Under no circumstance should you ever use a straight needle, always use a winged infusion set (butterfly needle). Here is a rule of thumb, if the vein to be drawn is below the antecubital fossa always use a butterfly needle.

Wrist/Hand: Drawing blood form the hand or wrist should always be your last resort for several reasons. First, the veins tend to rollover making it more difficult to insert the needle into the vein and there is a greater chance for a hematoma to occur, not to mention it is much more painful.

When drawing blood from the wrist it it important to stay away from the radial side of the wrist, as the radial artery could accidently be punctured. Several veins can be drawn from the hand they are; the top of the hand, along the thumb and between the fingers. Under no circumstances should you ever use a straight needle on the hand or wrist as this can cause damage, only use a butterfly needle.

Steps to a complete and successful venipuncture procedure:

Before we discuss the steps of a complete venipuncture procedure you need to be aware that there is no room for error. The procedure must me complete and precise from the time you greet the patient to completing the lab slip. What this also means there are "NO SHORT CUTS" in phlebotomy.

First and foremost, the procedure can be an intimidating experience for many patient's. I have never met a patient who was happy to have a needle put into their arm, it is for this reason the way you introduce yourself fron the very beginning is so vital. Keeping the patient calm from the beginning with youur excellent phlebotomy skills will greatly build a strong rapport between you and the patient. Let's now go through the steps from the beginning, "the waiting room" because this is where it all begins.

The Greeting: Some facilities may not allow calling out for a patient by first and last name simply because of patient privacy. However calling the patient by last name is permissable. For example Mr. or Ms. Smith. When the patient answers your call, greet them with a smile and eye contact. Welcome the patient and introduce yourself. For example; Good morning Mr/Ms Smith, my name is Anthony and I am your phlebotomist, please follow me to the lab. Once you have introduced yourself proceed to the blood drawing station and begin the identification process by asking the patient to spell his/her first and last name along with their date of birth. If any of the information on the lab requisition be incorrect it must be corrected before the procedure begins. Some labs also require that the phlebotomist ask the patient to review and initial the lab slip prior to beginning the procedure. Remember, the greeting along with proper identification is the foundation to building a

strong rapport between you and the patient, this is of course with your
excellent phlebotomy skills.

Explain the procedure: Explaining the procedure is just as important
as the greeting. Make the patient aware of the procedure you are about
to perform, this is especially true when performing a venipuncture on
pediatric patients. Explaining the procedure will also help the patient
understand the procedure and shows the patient you are a professional.

Place the tourniquet: The purpose of the tourniquet in phlebotomy
is to allow pressure to build up in the veins, allowing you to palpate
the vein and allows easier insertion of the needle. It is also important
to remember that the tourniquet cannot remain on the arm no longer
than one minute. The reason is after one minute has passed, hemolyses
can occur can occur causing the results of the test to become altered and
void ultimately affecting the patients well being. The doctor and the
patient count on you to perform your phlebotomy skills with precision.

Palpate the site: The purpose of palpating the site is to feel for a
suitable vein. I have often stated to my students, never go by what you
see but rather, go by what you feel, therefore, you must master the
sense of touch. When palpating a vein, you are feeling for spring like
action. Think of a rubber band, a good rubber band when stretched,
will snap back into it's original position. This is what you are feeling
for, when you press down on the vein it will bounce back, this will give
you an indication that you have found a good vein. If the vein feels
hard, this may be an indication the vein is sclerosed (hardened). A
sclerosed vein may have scar tissue due to possible over use of the vein.
If a vein feels like a string it may be a nerve and if punctured, could
cause extreme pain and sometimes numbness to the area. Should you
have any doubt about what you feel, always ask for a second opinion by
asking a coworker with more experience.

Remove the tourniquet: As mentioned, the tourniquet can only remain on the arm for no longer than one minute due the the possibility of hemolysis occuring.

Clean the puncture site: The site should be cleaned in a circular motion, beginning from the center working outwards bringing dirt away two to three inches from the puncture site. Never clean the site using an up and downward motion because this will only bring the dirt back to the puncture site which can potentially cause an infection. Only use approved alcohol wipes or povidone-iodine for blood cultures.

Prepare materials: The purpose of preparing your materials at this point is because until you have palpated the vein, you will not know whether to prepare a straight needle or butterfly needle. Therefore preparing the needle in advance will cause you to have prepared a needle you may not be able to use which must be discarded. Other material you are preparing is gauze, bandage, gloves, and tubes in proper order of draw.

Place on gloves: Some phlebotomists like to place gloves on at the very beginning. However, palpating a site with gloves on can be difficult, especially if the vein is deep or small. The gloves should be snug and most importantly, the gloves should cover the entire hand. Under no circumstance should you ever tear a piece of the glove for the sole purpose of repalpating a vein. This is when a phlebotomist tears the index finger portion of the glove to repalpate the site after the site has been cleaned. So what is wrong with this method? You have just palpated the site, cleaned the site just to retouch the site with your bare finger, now the site needs to be recleaned because of cross contamination. Remember, tearing a piece of the glove off is no different than not wearing a glove at all not to mention it's an OSHA violation.

Place the tourniquet: At this point the tourniquet can be placed on the arm. As a reminder, the tourniquet cannot remain on the arm no longer than one minute to prevent hemolysis.

Insert the needle: Always insert the needle with the bevel facing up. The way to thel the bevel is facing up is you will see the lumen (the opening of the needle). Glide the needle at a 45 degree angle and with the free hand insert and remove the test tubes. Never under any circumstance should you ever switch hand once the needle is inserted into the vein as the needle could shift and could cause pain to the patient, possibly causing a hematoma. To view proper needle insertion go to www.Phlebotomyfundamentals.com and click on venipuncture procedures.

Insert needle: Inserting the needle into the vein, you are now ready to begin inserting the test tube for blood collection. With you free hand, insert the test tubes in the proper order of collection. Remember under no circumstance should you ever switch hands.

Remove the tourniquet: With your free hand, remove the tourniqurt. This will release the pressure on the vein. Failing to remove the tourniquet prior to removing tube and needle can cause the a hematoma, therefore, always remove the tourniquet prior to removing the test tube. And as a reminder, hemolyses can occur if the tourniquet is on the arm longer than one minute.

Remove the test tube: The test tube should always be removed before the needle, the racational for this is if the test tube remains in the adaptor, blood form the tube can escape from the lumen of the needle. Once youe have collected all the test tubes needed, glide the needle out and with your free hans apply th gauze. Never place the gauze prior to removing the needle in the arm, pressing gauze down with the needle in the arm can cause the needle to bear down further into the patients arm and cause injury to the patient.

Apply bandage: The venipuncture is not complete until the bandage is placed on the venipunture site. Therefore, it is important that the patient always leave your facility with a bandage upon completing the procedure. Should a patient refuse a bandage, explain to them the reason which is the purpose of the bandage is to protect them from infection. If the patient is on a blood thinner such a wafarin (coumadin), they should never leave the lab without a bandage. In fact, you should place extra gauze and extra tape and ask the patient to keep the bandage on the arm for a least ten minutes. Some facilities require that a patient on blood thinners remain in the waiting area for a minimum of ten minutes before leaving the lab. If the site has not stopped bleeding after ten minutes, you should notify your supervisor or manager because a medical condition could be present which may require immediate attention.

Label the specimen: After placing the gauze on the venipuncture site and before placing the bandage on the patient, you should label the specimens in fron of the patient. The reason is so the patient observes you placing the labes on the specimen this also allows the patient to keep pressure on the site before placing the the bandage.

Thank the patient: Thanking the patient after the procedure solidifies the connection between you and the patient. It also shows the patient that you are a true professional and the feeling the patient will have about you as their phlebotomis will be remarkable because you will have established a great rapport with the patient, therefore, the patient may have a less sense of fear the next visit to the lab.

Lets recap the steps to a complete venipuncture.

1. Greet the patient
2. Explain the procedure
3. Place the tourniquet
4. Palpate the site
5. Remove the tourniquet
6. Clean the puncture site (in a circular motion in an inward outward motion)
7. Prepare materials
8. Place on gloves

9. Place on tourniquet
10. Insert needle (bevel up)
11. Remove tourniquet
12. Remove test tube
13. Apply gauze
14. Label specimens
15. Apply bandage
16. Thank patient

Always remember, that handwashing using OSHA standards must always be performed before and after any patient related procedure.

To view the entire venipuncture procedure go to www.phlebotomy fundamentals.com and click on venipuncture procedure.

Capillary Puncture
(Fingerstick)

A capillary puncture, often referred to as a fingerstick, is ordered when a small amount of blood is required such as a blood glucose test for diabetes or when obtaining blood from the heel of a newborn, although most facilities may not have you draw blood from an infant immediately until you have been properly trained. Should you work in a faciliity which obtains blood from infants or children, it is recommended that you ask to observe and to be cross trained. The ability to draw blood from children and infants is a great asset to add to your resume.

Capillary puncture: The following steps to a complete capillary puncture are as follows:

The greeting: As previously mentioned, the greeting is the most important ingredient prior to beginning any procedure. You should always greet the patient by callling out their last name for example, Mr/Ms Smith. Afterwords, with eye contact, introduce yourself. Upon entering the lab, ask the patient to verify their name and date of birth. If the patient has a wrist band, you should verify the name and date of birth. If the name or date of birth is incorrect either on the lab requisition or wrist band, you should stop the procedure and correct the information before continuing the procedure.

Explain the procedure: Explain to the patient that you willl be performing a fingerstick and that only a small amount of blood is needed.

Prepare material: Prepare all material needed for a complete capillary puncture. These items are:

- 2X2 gauze
- Lancet
- Alcohol wipe
- Collection tube
- Bandage

Place on gloves: As mentioned previously, gloves must be worn prior to handling specimens.

Prepare site for collection: When preparing the site, make sure the fingers are warm. If the fingers are cold, place a heat pack on the fingers for one minute, this will cause blood to circulate to the finger, this will cause the blood to flow out easily upon puncturing the finger. Puncturing a finger which is cold will clot immediately after the puncture.

Site Selection: The best fingers to use during a caplillary puncture are either the great finger or the ring finger. This is because there is greater circulation in these fingers and they are also easier to grip. Avoid using the index finger because it is more likely to be calloused, therefore, attempting to puncturing the index finger will be difficult. Also, avooid using the little finger because the skin is thin making the puncture painful.

Clean the site: Clean the finger using alcohol prep pads and allow the site to dry before puncturing the site. Not alloing the site to dry prior to the puncture can caue the alcohol to contaminated the specimen. This will cause the test to become void and the patient will need to be redrawn.

Puncture the site: Puncture the fleshy part of the finger, the fleshy part is on either side of the finger closest to the center. Do not puncture puncture parallel with the grooves (whorls) because the blood will run down the finger, instead, draw perpendicular with the grooves, this will cause the blood to come out in beads (drops) making it easier to colllect the specimen.

Collect the specimen: Upon puncturing the site, wipe off the first drop of blood because the first drop is contaminated with excess tissue and fluid, this can cause the test to be altered. After wiping off the first drop of blood, collect the specimen in the container provided by the lab. Never milk the finger during the collection because this can cause excess tissue to enter the specimen. Therefore, gently squeeze the finger and collect each bead of blood until the container is fill. Afterwords, gently invert the container to mix the anticoagulant with the blood. Never shake the container because hemolysis can occur.

Place gauze and label specimen: Upon successful completion of the fingerstick, place the gauze on the finger and label the specimen. Always label the specimen in front of the patient, this will allow the site to clot properly and the patient is observing you label the specimen.

Place bandage: Always place a bandage before allowing the patient to leave. If the patient refuses the bandage, explain to the patient the purpose of the bandage is to protect the site from infecton.

Never perform a capillary puncture on the fingers on infants because the needle can strike the bone causing an infection. Let's now look into proper capillary puncture on infants and young children.

Performing skin punctures of young children and infants is the preferred method because the veins are small and damage to the tissue and veins can occur. One of the most common tests performed on youn children and infants is phenylketonuria (PKU).

Infants: The recommended site for a skin puncture on infants is on the plantar surface of the heel. Let's now look at the steps of a complete skin puncture on infants.

- Identify the patient either by name braclet (if in hospital) or by asking the parent to identify the infant.
- Warm the heel for two to three minutes, this will allow blood to circulate and allow easier collection.
- Clean the site thoroughly and allow the site to dry. Not allowing the site to dry completely will cause the blood to not bead corretly making it difficult to collect.

- Prepare a 2mm lancet and gauze and bandage.
- Place on gloves
- Puncture the site on the plantar surface of the heel.
- Wipe off the first drop of blood. (The first drop may contain excess tissue fluids).
- Proceed to collect blood by using a little pressure and collect the beads of blood unto the microcontainer using a scooping motion. Collect each bead, and fill the microcontainer to the fill line. Upon completion, recap and invert the microcontainer eight to ten times gently to allow proper mixing of the blood with the additive. When collecting blood fron the finger or heel, you should never squeeze or message the site as this can cause excess tissue to enter the specimen along with the possibility of hemolysis to occur.
- Place gauze on the site.
- Label the specimen.
- Apply bandage to the site. To prevent choking, you should not apply a bandage on children under the age of two.
- Thank the parent of the child.
- Properly remove gloves and wash hands.
- Prepare specimen for transport.

As previously mentioned, as you begin your career, you may not be asked to immediately draw blood fron children or infants. However, It is strongly recommended that if you work in a facility that treats children and infants that you ask to observe as well as perform the procedure. This will help improve your skills as well make you more marketable.

Chapter 7

Additional Laboratory procedures

In this chapter we will discuss additional laboratory procedures you may be asked to perform. Some of these procedures you may learn either in class or cross trained in a facility. Some procedures may require you to become certified because of the nature of the procedure. Let's now explore some of these procedures beginning with Point of Care Tesing (POCT).

Point of Care Testing (POCT): Point of care testing brings laborarory testing to the patient. This can include bringing a hand held device such as a glucometer or portable EKG machine to the patients hospital bed or performing the procedure in the comfort of their home. Personnel who perform Point of Care Testing include, RN's, LPN's, medical assisants, nursing assistants, and phlebotomists. It is important to know that anyone performing POCT testing must be trained and recertified, this also includes understanding and performing proper quality control and maintenance procedures. Let's now look at some of the most common POCT procedures.

Glucose Testing: Glucose testing is the most common POCT procedure. It involves collecting a small amount of blood from the finger and placing the sample on to a special reagent strip which is inserted into a glucose monitoring device. To perform the test, follow the fingerstick procedure. Collect a drop of blood and apply it to the reagent strip. The results usually take thirty seconds to complete. Document the results upon completion of the test.

Pregnancy Testing: Pregnancy tests are used to detect the precence of Hunan Chorionic Gonadtropin (HCG) a hormone which is usually in the blood serum and urine approximately ten days after conception. When a physicain wants to rule out or confirm a pregnancy, a rapid pregnancy test may be ordered. Because there a several types of pregnancy test kits, it is importantt that you read and follow the instructions carefully.

Occult Blood (Guaiac): Occult blood tests also known as a Guaiac test is often performed during a physical examination or when a physician wants to rule out or confirm the presence of blood in the stool (feces) due to the possibility of disease of the digestive tract. The test includes the use of special kits. The test can be completed in the physicians office or at home. If an occult blood test is orderd, explain to the patient the test which has been ordered and the purpose of the test. Each kit should include three occult blood kits, and three sticks. The sticks resemble popsicle sticks, and are used to smear the stool onto a special reagent pad inside the card. Also provided with the kit are three toilet hats used to collect the stool. Explain to the patient, when they have a bowel movement, to collect a small amount of stool using the stick and to smear the stool on each pad inside of the card. Remember one card is used per **bowel movement.** To prevent a false positive result, instruct the patient to avoid eating foods such as spicy foods, radishes, or meat with blood in it. Upon receipt of the kits, you should log in the date and time of receipt. Place a drop of the special reagent fluid on each square. If blood is present in the feces there will be color change. Color changs should be reported to the ordering physicain immediaty.

Strep tests: When physicians need immediate strep test results He/She may order a rapid strep test. The entire test takes five minute from start to finish. Because of the sensitivity of the test, most laboratories will require certification. This is usually completed in the facility and will usually require yearly compentency review.

Urinalysis (UA): A urinalysis tests the physical and chemical components of the urine. When performing a urinalysis you are evaluating the following.

- Color: The normal color of urine is yellow/straw.
- Clarity/Transparency: Normal urine is clear.
- Cloudiness: Some causes of cloudy urine are: Bladder infection, Urinary Tract Infection (UTI), Kidney Stones.
- Odor: Normal urine does not have an odor. In fact the odor you smell is considered normal, this is because the urine has been sitting in the bladder until voiding (urinate). If urine has an odor of sugar or strong acid smell it should be reported immediately as this could be as sign of severe medical condition.

In most laboratories, a urine dipstick is performed. Urine dipsticks take three minutes from start to finish by using a narrow plastic strip. Each strip has colored squares which will react and change color. The urinalysis tests for the following:

- **Specific Gravity:** Specific gravity evaluates the bodies water volume and urine concentrate. The normal range for specific gravity is 1.005-1.030.
- **Leukocytes:** Leukocytes play a key role in the immune system. When leukocytes are present in the urine this could be an indication that an infection is present such a a urinary tract infection. Therefore, the normal range for leukocytes in urine should be negative. It should be noted as well that during female menstrual cycles, leukocytes may be present in the urine. This should be noted to the healthcare provider.

- Nitrites should not be present in the urine. Positive results may indicate the patient has a urinary tract infection (UTI). The presence of nitrites in the urine is called nitrituria

- **Urobilinogen:** Urobilinogen is the by product of bilirubin. Half of urobilinogen returns back to the liver while the rest is excreted through feces.. An increase of urobilinogen can be an indication of cirrhosis or hepatitis. Decreases levels of urobilinogen may be an indication of bileduct blockage and bileduct failure. Normal urobilinogen levels are 0 – 8 mg/dl.

- **Protein:** Protein is the building block for skin, muscle, hair, and tissues. There are over 10,000 types of proteins. One type is hemoglobin, an iron which contains protein that transports oxygen to the muscles via the bloodstream. The normal values for urine protein is 0 – 20 mg/dl. Excessive amounts of protein in the urine (Proteinuria) may be an indication of Dehydration, kidney failure, heart disease, urinary tract infection (UTI), overconsumption of protein.

- **ph:** The kidney's maintain normal acid-base balance through reabsorption of sodium and secretion of hydrogen and ammonium ions. High ph levels may be due to the kidneys not removing acids effeciently, urinary tract infection (UTI), kidney failure.

  Low ph levels may be due to; diarrhea, excessive acid in the body fluids, such as diabetic ketoacidosis a condition when the body uses fat a a source of energy instead of sugar (glucose) due to lack of insulin causing ketones, an acid build up in the body. Normal urine ph levels are 4.6 – 8.0.

- **Blood:** Blood in general is never present in urine. However, certain conditions may cause red blood cells to be present in blood such as:

Urinary Tract Infection (UTI): A Urinary Tract Infection (UTI) is a infection of any part of the urinary system. This could incude; the kidney's, urethra, ureters, or bladder.

Abrasion of the kidneys: This can be caused by kidney or bladder stones causing an irritation to the urinary tract. The blood may be gross (visible), or microscopic.

Trauma: Trauma to any portion of the urinary tract can cause bloody urine.

Medications: Medications such as aspirin, or coumadin may cause bloody urine.

Cancer: Cancer along the urinary tract may lead to bloody urine.

The term for blood in the urine is Hematuria.

- **Ketones:** The body produces a substance called ketones when the body breaks down fat for energy and therefore, are passed into the urine. A large amount of ketones in the urine may be a sign of a condition called diabetic ketoacidosis, which can lead to an intoxication of the bloodstream. Large amounts of ketones can lead to poisoning of the body which can lead to dehydration and swelling of the brain.

- **Bilirubin:** Bilirubin is a substance formed by the breakdown of red blood cells. Bilirubin is passed through the body through stool. The presence of bilirubin in urine nmay be an indication of a damaged liver or the flow of bile through the gallbladder is blocked.

- **Glucose:** Glucose is a sugar found in the blood. Normally glucose is never present in urine. The presence of glucose in urine may be an indication of uncontrolled diabetes, this is when sugar spills over into the urine. Other causes of glucose in the urine could be due to damaged kidneys or kidney disease.

- **Microscopic Analysis:** Upon collection of a urine sample in a sterile cup, the technician pipets some urine from the cup into a special tube. The tube is then placed into a centrifuge and spun allowing solid material (sediments) o settle to he bottom of the tube. The sediment is then spread across a slide and viewed under a microscope. The following may be seen on the slide:

- **Red Blood Cells (Erythrocytes) or White Blood Cells (Leukocytes):** Normally red blood cells or white blood cells are never found in urine. However, disease of the kidneys ureters or the bladder may cause blood in the urine. Running large distances such as a marathon or strenuous exercise can also cause blood in the urine. When white blood cells are present this may be an indication of an infection such as a Urinary Tract Infection (UTI) or kidney disease.

- **Crystals:** It is not uncommon to find a few crystals in healthy people, however, large amounts of certain types of crystals may indiate the presence of kidney stones.

- **Casts:** Some types of kidney disease may cause material called casts to form in the small tubes inn the kidneys and get flushed out into the urine. Casts can be made up of protein, waxy or fatty substances, or red or white blood cells. Depending on the type of cast can help in determine whatbtype of kidney disease is present.

- **Squamous Cells:** Squamous cells are flat scaly cells and are found on the top layer of the skin, tissue that lines the passageway of the digestive tract, or the inside lining of organs such as the bladder. Therefore, the specimen may not be considered pure, however, the phisician may order the patient leave a new urine sample.

- **Bacteria, Yeasts or Parasites:** Normally, there are no bacteria, yeast cells or paracites in urine. If there is a presence, this may indicate the presence of an infection.

- **Clean-Catch Midstream collection:** This type of test can be ordered as a routine test or when a patient complains of frequent urination (polyuria) or painful urination (dysuria). The following steps must be completed properly, or the test will be inaccurate.

For male patients:

- Explain the procedure to the paient.
- Explain to the patient to wash his hands prior to removing the lid from the cup.
- Explain tto the patiient not to place his hands inside the cup as this can cause contamination.
- Ask the patient to retract the foreskin, if present and to clean the head of the penis with the medicated towelettes.
- Begin urinating (voiding) into the urinal. After the urine has flowed for a couple of seconds Collect the specimen into the cup provided and proceed to collect about 60ml of urine.
- Upon filling the cup, finish urinating into the toilet.
- Explain to the patient, upon completion to replace and tighten the lid and to leave the cup in a deginated place.

For female patients:

- Explain the procedure to the patient.
- Explain the the patient to wash her hands priior to removing the lid from the cup.

- Explain to the patient not to place her hands inside the cup as this can cause contamination.
- Explain to the patient to hold apart the the genital fold with one hand and with the other hand clean the area surrounding the urethra with medicated towelettes. Explain to clean the area from front to back so that bacteria from the anus is not wiped across the urethra.
- Ask the patient to hold back the genital folds during urination.
- Ask the patient to begin urinating into the toilet.
- After a few seconds, ask the patient to begin urinating into the cup.
- Remind the patient to avoid getting pubic hair, toilet paper, or menstrual blood or anything else as this can cause the results to become altered.
- After the patient has collected the sample ask her to finish urinating into the toilet.
- Ask the patient to replace and tighten the lid and return the specimen in the desinated area.

- **24 Hour urine protein test:** A 24 hour urine is ordered to check the function of the kidneys to detect kidney disease such as proteinuria (excessive amount of protein in the urine).

  The specimen is collected over a 24 hour period in a container provided by the lab. The specimen should remain in a cool area until the container is brought back to the lab for analysys.

- **Reasons a 24 hour urine protein test are ordered:** The purpose of the test is to detect the amount of protein in the urine. Protein levels can rise due to factors such as stress, infeection, and excessive exercise all of which are generally temprorary. However, excessive amounts protein (proteinuria) could signify serious kidney damage. Proteinuria is caused by the following conditions.

- Daibetes
- Bladder cancer
- Urinary Tract Infection (UTI)
- Congestive Heart failure (CHF)
- The use of medications that can damage the kidneys
- Lupus (an inflammatory autoimmune disease)
- Kidney infection
- Hypertension (high blood pressure)
- Polycystic kidney disease (cysts on the kidneys)
- Multiple Myeloma (cancer of the plasma cells)
- Glomerulonephritis (inflammation of the blood vessels in kidneys)
- Heavy metal poisoning

Prepaing the patient for a 24 hour protein urine test::

- Explain the procedure to the patient.
- Give the patient the container and specimen hat to collect the urine.
- Instruct the patient to begin collecting the specimen with the exception of first morning urination, and begin timing each collection.
- Refrgerate or place specmen into a cooler with some ice to preserve the specimen.
- Instruct the patient to collect the last specimen in the morning and transpot the specimen to the lab as soon as possible.

Catheterized Urine Specimen: Patients who have difficulty urinating (voiding) will have a sterile catheter inserted. This is done by inserting a sterile catheeter throuh the urethra into the bladder. In some cases, a patient may already have a catheter inserted, this could be due to urinary incontinence, urinary retention, or bedridden patients. It is also important to understand some of the complications of catheterization.

- Urunary tract or kidney infection
- Uretheral injury

- Blood infections (Septicemiia)
- Blood in the urine (Hematuria)
- Bladder stones

Types of catheters:

- **Straight-Single use catheter:** This type of catheter has a small opening (Lumen)
- Coude (curved) catheter: This type of catheter has a curved rounded tip and is generally used on males with enlarged prostates which can cause the urethra to become partilly blocked. This usuallly occurs in older males.
- **2-way Foley Catheter:** This type of catheter has an inflatable balloon which encircles th tip near the lumen.
- **3-way catheter:** This type of catheter has 2 or three lumens that encircle the body of the catheter. One lumen drains the urine through the catheter into the collection bag. The second lumen contains sterile water used to inflate the catheter and deflate the balloon. The third catheter when needed, is used to instill medications into the bladder or can also be a route for continuous bladder irrigation.

Semen Analysys: In some cases, a provider may order a semen analysis. This type of test is used to detect the effectiveness of a vasectomy (sterilization) or to assess fertility. Semen samples are collected in sterile conatiners. It is important to understand and to instruct the patient not to collect the specimen from a condom because many condoms contain spemicides which kill sperm. After the collection the specimen shoould be kept warm and delivered to the lab immediately.

Miscellaneous tests:

The following tests are not performed by the phlebotomist, but understanding the purpose and how the specimen is collected will give you a better prospective of the test. It should be noted that all body cavity fluids are collected in a sterile container and in most cases delivered to the lab stat and analyzed immediately.

Cerebrospinal Fluid (CSF): Cerebrospinal fluid is a clear and colorless fluid that circulates within the cavities which surround the brain and spinal cord. CSF specimens are obtained by physicians and often collected through the spine also known as a spinal puncture or spinal tap. Some tests performed on the spine include:

- Chloride
- Total Protein
- Glucose
- Cell Counts

Amniotic fluid: Amniotic fluid surrounds the fetus in the uterus and is normally clear, colorless to pale yellow fluid. The specimen is collected by inserting a needle into the abdominal wall into the fetus. The name of the procedure is called transabdominal amniocentesis. The fluid after 15 weeks of gestation. The purpose of the test is to monitor fetal development and to detect geneic defects through chromosome analysis. Amniotic fluid must always be collected in a sterile container, be protected from light and dellivered to the lab immediately. Some risk factors of an amniocentesis include:

- **Leaking amniotic fluid**- in most cases fluid loss is small and stops within one week.
- **Miscarriage**- A slight risk of a miscarriage can occur during the second trimester about .6 percent. However, amniocentesis performed prior to 15 weeks have a higher risk of pregnancy loss.
- **Rh Sensitization**- Although rare, an amniocentesis may cause the baby's bllod cells to leak into the mother's bloodstream. If the mother's is Rh negative and has not developed Rh positive antibodies, the mother willl be injected with a blood product called Rh immune globulin after an amniocentesis.. This will

prevent the mother's body from producing Rh antibodies which can damage the baby's red blood cells.

- **Needle injury**- Because the baby may move during an amniocentesis, there is a rare chance that an arm or leg becomes punctured causing injury.
- Infection- Uterine infection can occur following an amniocentesis but is very rare.
- Infection transmission- If the mother is infected with HIV/ AIDS or Hepatitis C the infection might be transmitted to the baby during an amniocentesis.

Nasopharyngeal (NP) culture- Nasopharyngeal cultures are collected by inserting a cotton tipped swab into the nasopharynx. The swab is gently rotated and then gently removed and placed into a transport media and ssnt to the lab for analysis. An NP is ordered by the provider to detect microorganisms that cause:

- Pertussis (Whooping cough)
- Meningitis
- Pneumonia
- Diphtheria

As mentioned, asking to observe any procedure will help you to appreciate the importance of the test and how very important it is that you not only handle the specimen carefully, but making sure the specimen is brought to the lab with extreme important as is with all specimens.

Chapter 8

Specimen handeling/Quality control/Quality Assurance

In this next chapter, we will be discussing in detail the importance of quality assurance and specimen handeling. We will also discuss the roll of the Joint Commission on Accreditation of Healthcare Organizations (JCAHO), Total Quality Management (TQM), dimensions of performance, and the ten step monitoring and evaluation process. You as a healthcare professional have a moral and ethical duty to the patient, not to mention that the patient and the provider rely on your expertise and ability to perform your duties with precision. Let's begin.

Joint Commission on Accreditation of Healthcare Organizations (JCAHO):

Let's first understand that JCAHO is a nongovernmental agency who which is a key player in bringing continuous quality improvement (CQI) to the healthcare facility and is a national accreditation body for hospitals. There role is to set standards for hospitals, healthcare facilities and services. In 1994, JCAHO required that all healthcare facilities, hospitals, and their services have an institution-wide total quality management (TQM) and continuous quality improvement plan in place. What this means is that all facilities and their deparments must have ongoing evaluations of patient care and performance accountability. Let's now examine performance accountability. They are doing the right thing and doing the right thing well.

Doing the right thing:

- Efficacy- The ability to produce the intended outcome of a procedure or treatment related to the patient's condition. For example, the ability to show the desired outcome(s).
- Appropriateness- Properly performing a specific test, procedure, or service that meets the patient's needs. For example, tests which are relevant to the patient's clinical needs.

Doing the right thing well:

- **Availability**- The ability to perform a procedure, test or service to the patient who needs it. In other words, making sure that appropriate care can meet the patients needs.
- Timeliness- the time in which a procedure, test treatment, or service is provided to the patient when it is most benificial.
- **Effectiveness**- To provide tests, procedures, treatments, and services to the patient in a correct manner and to achieve the best projected outcomes for the patient.
- **Continuity**- Services provided to the patient in which care is coordinated amongst other services, practitoners, and providers over time.
- Safety- To the patient (and others) in which the risk of an intervention and risk in the care enviroment are reduced to the patients's and other's, including the providers.
- **Efficiency**- The relationship between the outcomes and the resourses used to care for the patient the best way possible.
- **Respect and caring**- In which the patient or designee involved in his or her own decisions and to those providing services do so with utmost sesitivity and respect for the patient's needs and expectations.

Total Quality Management (TQM): Total quality management stresses the importance of improvement rather than just being satified with meeting the minimum standards. In other words, seeking better ways to making a continuous effort to improve services. So whether you work in a clinical setting or in a healthcare facility, quality is always the major priority.

- Ensuring that services, care, and outcome are always athe their best.
- Understanding whou your patient's are and committ to serving their need and providing them with the best possible care.
- You should always seek to improve. Afterall, anything can be improved on.
- Focusing on making the process easier and to better understand the customers needs.
- Ensuring that each patient is informed on how they're doing.
- Ensuring quality is aways a priority.
- Ensuring the job is done right the first time by seeking ways to eliminate the complexity of the job.
- Continuing to educate and improve by attending trainings and seminars.
- Focusing on teamwork and following protcols established by the facility
- Focusing on keeping the mission statement simple so that all parties can stay focused on doing the right thing.

Quality Assurance: In the late 1980's JCAHO developed a 10-step monitoring and evaluation process used to assess the appropriateness of care. The purpose of the 10-step rule to to assist the healthcare facility in putting together and implement a plan where all departments are given the responsibilty to perform high quality performance. Generally a quality improvement committee is formed and meet on a frequent basis, usually quartely. There responsibility is to:

- Monitor routine activities
- Evaluate clinical outcomes

- Review incident reports
- Conducts problem- focused studies in an effort to identfy practices which fall below quality standards.

Members of the quality improvement committee include the following:

- Represenative from clinical personnel.
- Represenative from the administrative committee.
- Quality improvement coordinator.
- Risk manager.

The 10-step monitoring and evaluation process:

- Assign responsibility.
- Delineate scope of care.
- Identify important aspects of care.
- Identify indictors related to these aspects of care.
- Establish thresholds for evaluation related to the indicators.
- Collect and organize data.
- Evaluate care when thresholds are reached.
- Take actions to improve care.
- Assess the effectiveness of actions and document improvements.
- Communicate relevant information to the organization-wide quality assurance program.

Quality Control (QC): Quality control is a procedure or set of procedures that are followed during any given procedure. This involves in monitoring all operational procedures from the person performing a particular procedure such as phlebotomy and EKG to the devices used to perform a procedure. For example, prior to beginning a glucose test, the phlebotomist or the person responsible should always QC the glucometer. This assures the device is working properly by testing the device using high and low controls. If the controls show within normal range the person performing the QC should sign ths control log a normal and the device can be used. However, should the results be out of range, the person performong the QC should note the problem in the log and notify the supervisor so the device can be brought for recalibration. Under no circumstances should any diagnostic device be used if not properly functioning. Always report the problem and use a device which is properly functioning.

Another example of quality control is ensuring that the phlebotomist performing the procedure is meeting the standards. This is accomplished by the supervisor who oversees the the phlebotomist or any healthcare professional. Generally, on a yearly basis, all healthcare professionals are required to undergo a compentency test in all areas of their skill levels.

Let's now examine quality control in the clinical setting.

Patient Identification: As mentioned previously, proper patient identification is the most important form of quality control. Using a two method identification will ensure that you are collecting a specimen on the correct patient. This is by asking the patient to say their name and date of birth. Should either one be incorrect, or if the date of birth is off, even by one number then you must stop and have the information corrected prior to beginning. Explain this to the patient and let them know it is for their safety. Under no circumstances should you correct their name or date of birth by crossing out the information and writing in the correct information. In most labs today, lab requisitions and labels have bar codes and any discrepancy can result in a mislabeled specimen which could result in having the patient come in and having their labs redrawn. This leads to longer wait time for the results and patient frustration.

Labeling: Just like patient identification, the label must be correct. Any inaccuracies must be corrected prior to performing any procedure. Specimens sent to the laborarory with incorrect information will be discarded and noted as a mislabeled specimen.

Evacuated Tubes: Just like proper patient identification, proper validation of evacuated tubes is important. This means checking the expiration date. Tubes which have expired should be discarded. Using tubes which have expired can cause dilution of the sample or the tube may not fill completely. Therefore, prior to opening up a new lot of evacuated tubes, check the date of expiration. And when restocking, always put the new tubes on the bottom, this will eliminate any chance of tubes becoming expired.

Control checks: Depending on the device, control checks are performed on a daily weekly, or monthly basis, for example, a glucometer is checked daily before the clinic opens where the eyewash station is checked on a weekly basis. In fact, JCAHO who accredates a facility requires the facility to show documentation. Equipment which has failed a control check, must be tagged and sent to be repaired

Procedure Manual: JCAHO requires that a procedure manual (Lab Manual) be available. The manual provides information regardng each test performed in the lab. JCAHO, also requires laborarory procedure manuals be updated on a yearly basis. Information provided includes.

- Purpose of the procedure
- Specimen type and collection method
- Equipment and supplies required
- Detailed step-by-step procedure
- Limitations and variables of the method
- Corrective actions
- Method validation
- Normal values and references

It's important to know the procedure manual is updated on a frequent basis and any notifications of any changes are also brought to the nursing staff. Also the procedure manual is a quality assurance document and it's intent is to assure that the lab adheres to the national standard of good practice. Along with the procedure manual, JCAHO also requires all laborarories to show documentation of quality control checks. Special forms are used to record equipment checks and genrally are performed by the phlebotomist on a routine basis. Some of the equipment which must routinely be checked are the glucometer, Centrifuge, urine analyzer, refrigerator temperatures. Besides checking equipment, control checks are also performed on collections tubes, guaiac test cards, control solutions and control strips. All facilities will require you to undergo quality control training and on a yearly basis, perform a compentency review. This form is signed by you and the person performing the training and the yearly review and kept in your employee file.

Specimen Handling: To maintain specimen integrity, all specimes must be handled with importance. Every facility establishes specimen handling procedures and must always be followed. These procedures not only maintain the integrity of the specimen but also protects the person handling the specimen from accidental exposure to potentially infectious diseases. Every facility which handles patient specimens establishes specimen handling tecniques and should always be followed. In fact, the Centers for Disease Control (CDC) has written guidelines on how specimens should be handled. The guidelines are also enforced by the Occupational Safety and Health Administration (OSHA). Let's now examine some other specimen handling procedures.

Transporting Specimens: Specimens can be transported in different ways. Nonetheless, whichever way a specimen is transported, it must be with extreme care. For instance, blood specimens should be transported with the top facing up which aids in clot formation of serum tubes and prevents contact with the tube stopper. Blood which has contact with a stopper can potentially become contaminated, this can also contribute to aerosol which is a fine mist of the specimen during stopper removal. Specimens blood or nonblood can also be transported through a pheumatic tube system. This type of delivery requires the specimen to be protected from shock and to prevent hemolysis from occuring. specimens should be transported in a leak-proof container. Specimens delivered to the lab from an off-site location should be transported with extra care because the specimen may be subjected to extreme conditions such as hot and cold. Therefore the specimen should be protected. For instance in hot weather the specimens should be In a cooler to prevent the inaccurate results. Some specimens require additional special handling.

Specimens that need to be chilled: Chilling the specimen slows down the metabolic process. Therefore, placing the specimen in a continer with crushed ice and water or large cubes of ice without water will provide adequate cooling. However, you should be mindful not to place any specimen in direct contact with a solid piece of ice, this can cause freezing resulting in hemolysys. Examples of tests which require chilling are ammonia, blood gas, and lactic acid. You should always consult with the lab manual or the main lab for proper specimen delivery.

Specimens that need to be kept warm: Some specimens require that the specimen be kept warm while it is being trasported, This can be done by wrapping the specimen in a heel warmer, this will keep the specimmen near body temperature (37 degrees celsius). An example of a test which needs to stay warm is a cryoglobulin test.

Specimens requiring protection from light: Some tests require the light not be present the blood components can break down. Therefore, after collect the specimen, you should wrap the specimn in allumium foil, thiis will aid in the prevention of light from entering. Some specimens which require no light are; vitmin B12, carotene. As mentioned previously, if you are not sure, always check with your supervisor or lab manual for proper specimen handeling.

Specimen Delivery: Ideally, specimens should be sent to the lab within 45 minutes to one hour

Generally, on site labs such a a hospital setting, specimes can be sent by a pneumatic tube system. This type of system propels tubes via compressed air or by partial vacuum to its destination. Another form of deliver is through an in housd carrier service. Should the specimens come from an off site lab, the specimen is first cenrifuged and picked up by a courier service and sent to the hosptal lab for analysis. In some cases, specimens are ordered "Stat" (immediately), these type of specimens regardless if the lab on or off site the specimen is sent immediately. These type of specimens always take priority over all specimens.

Specimen Processing: All laborarories have a specimen processing department also known as central processing. In this department, specimens are received, triaged (prioritized) and prepared for testing. Upon receiving the specimen, labs are accessioned (logged in), and sorted. Labs are then sent to the appropriate department for centrifugation (if required) and tested. As mentioned previously, prior to sending the specimen, always check the labels and the lab requisition. Sending specimens with mislabeled tubes, will cause a delay in processing and can cause patient frustration. And as always, remember to use proper protective equipment pror to specimen collecton and delivery. OSHA requires all persons handeling body fluids must wear protective equipment such as a mask, goggles, faceshields and gloves.

Chapter 9

Vitals and additional Point of Care Tests

Vitals are an important piece to a patients well being. Anyone who has patient contact especially in the clinical setting should have the ability to perform vitals. Vitals include, Blood pressure, pulse respiration, and oxygen saturation (O2 sats). Although, some clinics may use automated machines which perform blood pressure and pulse, being able to perform vitals the manual way with the exception of O2 saturation is extremly important. I have always taught my students the manual way for the single most important reason and that is manually performing vitals is more accurate. But first, you must know what you are performing. Let's now examine patient vitals.

Blood Pressure (BP): Blood pressures are measured by using the brachial artery located in the upper arm and the device used is a sphigmomanometer or know as a BP cuff. The results are measured in millimeters and are read from a gauge. But before a blood pressure can be performed let's understand the significance of blood pressure.

According to the American Heart Association (AHA) the optimal blood pressure range for adults is less than 120/80 mm Hg.

Blood Pressure Ranges: The following blood pressure ranges has been established by the American Heart Association:

- **Normal Blood Pressure:** Adult patients with a blood pressure reading of less than 120/80 mm/ Hg are catagorized as having a normal blood pressure. Generally, patients with a normal blood pressure, have healthy diets and exercise.
- **Prehypertension:** Adult patients with prehypertension blood pressure have a consistant pressure of 120-139/ 80-89 mm Hg. Patients with prehypertension can develop hypertension. They should seek the quidance of their health are provider to help maintain a healthy lifestyle.
- **Hypertension Stage 1:** Adult patients with Stage 1 hypertension have a consistant pressure of 140-159/90-99 mm Hg. Patients diagnosed with stage 1 hypertension are likely to be prescribed blood pressure medication and advised to change their daily lifestyle habits.
- **Hypertension Stage 2:** Adult patients with stage 2 hypertension have a consistant pressure of 160/100 mm Hg. During this stage of hypertension the provider is likely to prescribe high blood pressure medications along with lifestyle changes.
- **Hypertensive Crisis:** This type of blood pressure is when the pressure is greater than 180/110 mm Hg and requires emergency medical attention. In some cases the provider may order an EKG while they are awaiting for emergency responders to arrive.

Blood Pressure Readings:

Systolic Pressure: Systolic pressure is the top number of the BP reading and refers to the amount of pressure on the arteries during contraction.

Diastolic Pressure: Diastolic pressure is the bottom number of the BP and refers to when the heart muscle is between beats.

You should also know that the systolic blood pressure is typically given more attention to patients over 50 because of the risk factor for cardiovascular disease. Increased systolic blood pressure also rises with age, this is due to long term build-up of plaque and the stiffening of the large arteries.

Blood pressure measurement:

Any healthcare professional who has direct contact with a patient must follow proper steps when performing a blood pressure. It can not be stressed enough the importance of accurately performing and recording a blood pressure. Let's begin.

- Ask the patient if they consumed caffenated beverages or smoked In the last 30 minutes. These can cause a false high blood pressure reading. Should they have smoked or consumed a caffenated beverage, note this in the patient chart and inform the provider.
- Have the patient sit calmly for about five minutes. This can be done while assessing the patient.
- The patient's arms should be bare. Avoid placing the cuff over clothing. Placing a cuff over clothing can cause a tourniquet effect. Studies have also shown, that placing the cuff over clothing can impact the systolic blood pressure anywhere from 10-50 mm Hg.
- Support the patient's arm by placing it on a firm surface at heart level. You can also hold the patient's arm if no surface to place the arm is available.
- Instruct the patient to refrain from talking while you are taking their blood pressure. This cn cause the blood pressure to increase slightly.
- Use the apppropriate cuff size. For instance if the cuff is too small, the patient's systolic blood pressure can increase by 10 to 40 mm Hg.

- Snugly wrap the cuff around the bare arm. The cuff should also be centered two finger widths above the bend of the elbow.
- Make sure the anaroid meter is visable and facing you.
- Position the diaphragm od the stethoscope over the brachial artery. Under no circumstances should you place the stethoscope directly under the cuff. Placing the stethoscope directly under the cuff will put pressure against the diaphragm of the stethoscope making it difficult to hear the blood pressure.
- Record the blood pressure in increments of two. For example 120/80 mm Hg.

To View a complete Blood pressure, go to Phlebotomy fundementals. com and click on vitals.

Heart Rate: The heart rate also known as the pulse is the number of times the heart beats per minute. The average adult resting heart rate is 60 to 100 beats per minute. Patients who have are physically active often, have a lower heart rate because their heart muscle is conditioned. Therefore, the heart doesn't need to work as hard. Resting heart rates greater than 100 beats per minute means the heart muscle (Myocardium) needs to work harder to maintain bodily functions. You should also take note that other factors can affect the heart rate such as Beta-Blockers. Beta-Blockers such as Atenolol or metoprolol are used for irregular heartbeats (arrhythmia), high blood pressure (Hypertension), or after a heart attack (myocardial infarction). Beta-Blheart blockers, block the effects of stress hormones such as ad adrenaline also know as epinephrine.

Just like taking the patients blood pressure, the heart rate (pulse) must be properly taken. Make sure the patient has not had any caffenated beverages or smoked in the last 30 minutes. To take a resting pulse, find the radial pulse which is located on the thumb side of the wrist. Gently place two fingers on the artery. Do not put pressure on the artery because it will make it difficult to feel the artery. Upon feeling the artery, begin counting for 60 seconds. The purpose of taking it for 60 seconds, asisde for counting the beats per minute, you are also feeling for any irregularities such as skipped beats or rapid beats which should be noted in the patient's chart. Some facilites may permit taking the pulse for 30 seconds and times it by two, however, it should be noted that if you perform the 30 second method and you feel any irregularities, you should continue for the full 60 seconds. Under no circumstances should you use your thumb because it has it's own pulse.

Respiration: The respiration also known as the respiratory rate is the number of breaths a patient takes per minute. The normal adult respiration rate is 12 to 20 breaths per minute. The best way to count the patients respirations is to keep your fingers on the patients wrist as if you are taking their pulse and begin watching their chest rise and fall for 30 seconds and times it by two. One respiration consists of one inhalation and one expiration. You should not announce to the patient that you are about to take their respiration because they will alter the way they breath. Therefore, take the respiration along with the pulse, this is the best and most effective way to determine both vital signs.

To view a complete pulse and respiration in it's entirety, go to phlebotomy fundamentals.com and click on vitals.

Orthostatic Vitals signs: Orthostatic vital signs are a series of mesurements of the patients blood pressure and pulse. The vital signs are are taken with the patient in the supine position (laying down), sitting, and standing.

Performing orthostatic vitals: It's extremly important that ortostatic vitals are performed correctly and with precision. Orthostatic vitals are ordered when the patient comes in with signs and symptoms of orthostasis (lightheadedness), after a fall or when a patient is taking medications which may cause ortostasis and risk factors for falls.

Step-by-step procedure:

- Introduce youself.
- Explain the procedure.
- Wash hands.
- Instruct thee patient to to lie down in the supine position with the head flat for a minimum of 3 minutes.
- Measure the patient's blood pressure and pulse while in the supine position.
- Instruct the patient to sit for I minute. During this time, ask the patient if they feel dizzy or weak while in the sittting position.
- Measure the patient's blood pressure and pulse in the sitting position. If the patient shows symptoms of dizziness associated with the position change or has a blood pressure below 90/60, put the patient back in bed and notify the provider.
- Instruct the patient to stand, and ask if they feel dizzy or weak and note any changes. If the patient is unable to stand, have the patient sit upright with their legs dangling over the edge of the bed. Should the patient develop syncope (faint) of or shows signs of syncope developing, immediately lay the patient back in the supine position and notify the provider.
- If the patient shows no signs of dizziness or weakness, have the patient stand for 3 minutes. Support the patient's forearm at heart level for proper measurement. Measure he patient's blood pressure and pulse.
- Assist the patient back in bed and into a comportable position.
- Document the vital signs taken in every position and any pertinent information in the patient's medical record.

Pulse Oximetry: Pulse oximetry is a simple, and noninvasive procedure The device used is called a pulse oximeter. The oximeter, measures the amount of oxygen also known as oxygen saturation in the blood.

The pulse oximeter uses a device called a probe which compares and calulates oxygen rich hemoglobin and oxygen poor hemoglobin.

One side of the probe contains two different types of light, infrared and red. These lights are transmitted through the body's tissues to the light detector. Hemoglobin that contains a rich amount of oxygen absorbs more of the infrared light. On the other hand, hemoglobin that lacks oxygen absorbs more of the red light.

Located in the probe is a microprocessor that calculates the converts the information into a digital value. The value is determines the of oxygen carried in the blood.

Reasons for using a pulse oximeter: The pulse oximeter is used for a variety of reasons:

- During surgeries or other procedures that involve sedation and to make any adjustmennts of supplemental oxygen during the procedure.
- During routine examinations.
- Assess whether to adjust the amount of oxygen is needed.
- Patient's who have sleep apnea (an serious condition where breathing is interrupted).
- Heart Attack.
- Chronic Obsructive Pulmonary Disease (COPD).
- Lung Cancer
- Anemia
- Asthma
- Bronchitis
- Pneumonia
- Congestive Heart Failure (CHF)

How to properly use a pulse oximeter:

- Introduce youself.
- Verify the patient.
- Explain the procedure.
- Wash hands.

- Place probe on finger. (for best results, rest the patient's hand on their chest at heart level. This minimizes movment. Any type of movement can affect the reading.
- Record the measurement. A normal range is considered between 95%-100%. Any value below 95% should be brought to the provider's attention.

It should be noted that anything that absorbs light such as nail polish should be removed to avoid false low readings. Fingers should also be warm, cold fingers can cause poor blood flow which can cause the oximeter to make an error in it's reading.

Ear Irrigations: An ear irrigation aslo know as ear lavage is a procedure used to remove excessive earwax (Cerumen) or foreign material from the ear. A custom-designed Syrange with a nozzle attached to it is used to flush out excessive ear wax or foreign material. The syrange gently flushes using warm water.

Performing an ear irrigation:

- Introduce yourself
- Verify the patient.
- Wash hands
- Place on gloves
- Place the patient inn a comfortable position.
- Place towels and drapes on the patient's shoulder's.
- Place warm water with solution in a basin.
- Fill the syrange with with warm water and solution contained in the basin.
- As the patient to tilt their head slightly.
- Ask the patient to hold a clean basin under the ear.
- Gently, begin flushing the ear.
- With the opposite hand, pull the auricle to straighten the ear canal.

- Gently insert the syrange making sure not to go to deep and begin flushing
- Repeat irrigation per providers instructions
- Upon completion, blot the outer ear dry.
- Notify the provider the procedure is complete.
- Discard contents per OSHA regulations.

If the patient at any time during the irrigation complains of pain, stop the proceure and notify the provider.

Throat cultures: A throat culture or throat swab is used to determine whether the infection is viral or bacterial. The most common bacteria that causes strep throat is streptococcus pyogenes (Strep A streptococcus).

Step-by-step procedure:

- Introduce yourself.
- identify the patient by asking their name and date of birth.
- Explain the procedure.
- Wash hands.
- Place on gloves.
- Instruct he patient to tilt their head back slightly.
- With a wooden tongue depressor hold the tongue down. With the free hand, use a sterile cotton swab and gently swab the back of the throat. Be careful not to touch the uvula, lips or tongue due to possible contamination.

- Place swab into transport medium.
- Label sample and confirm patient's name and date of birth.
- Send specimen to lab for analysis.

It should be noted that many provider's perform a rapid strep test prior to sending a sample to the lab for analysis. The collection procedure is the same only this time the swab is placed in a specialized container for analysis. The procedure takes 5 minutes to complete. Because there ar different types of rapid strep test kits, you should read the instructions prior to performing the test. In fact, most clinics require an on site training for healthcare professionals who will be performing rapid strep tests.

Urine Pregnancy Test: Approximately 7-10 days after conception the developing placenta produces a glycoprotein hormone called Human Chorionic Gonadtropin (HCG). When the patient has missed the first menstrual period, the provider may order a urine pregnancy test.

Step-by-step procedure:

- Introduce yourself.
- Verify the patient by asking their name and date of birth.
- Provide the patient with a sterile urine cup.
- Upon receiving the urine sample, open a test cassette from the sealed pouch. As with any collection device, you should always check the expiration date prior to usage.
- Using a pipette, vertically transfer 3 drops of urine into the wall of the cassette.
- Wait for the red lines to appear.
- Read the results within 3-4 minutes.
- Interpret results: Negative-one red line appears on the control.
Positive-two red lines appear.
- Should the redline not appear on the control repeat the test.
- Record and provide results to the provider.

Clinics may require an on site training prior to performing any type of point of care testing.

To view urine pregnancy testing, go to phlebotomy fundementals.com and click urine pregnancy.

Chapter 10

Electrocardiography
(EKG/ECG)

The electrocardiography is an essential part in evaluating patients who are complaining of chest pain. The electrocardiogram is the front line diagnostic tool used to detect cardiac arrhythmias (abnormal heart rhythm). The healthcare provider relies on the technician performing the electrocardiogram. Therefore, it is not only important to understand the purpose of an electrocardiogram, but more importantly is to perform it with precision. But before we begin, let's understand where it all began.

Around 1901 a Dutch physician, Willem Einthoven invented the string galvanometer also known as the Einthoven galvanometer. The galvanometer is a instrument used to detect and measure electrical current. In fact the origianal galvanometer required 5 operators because it weighed around 600 pounds and it also needed water to cool the electromagnets. The prodecure was performed by having the patient sit and placing both arms and the left leg in seperate buckets of saline solution. The buckets acted as electrodes to conduct the current from the skins surface to a filament. The three limbs, produced what is know as Einthoven's triangle, a principal used even in today's EKG recordings. If you were wondering why the right leg was not placed in water, it's because the right leg acted as the ground. Even today, the right leg acts as the ground. In 1924 Einthoven was awarded the nobel prize in medicine.

Electrode placement: It cannot be emphasized enough that the correct placement of the electrodes (sensors) is a vital piece to recording the perfect EKG. Incorrect placement of the electrodes can result in a misdiagnosis. So let's look in detail what the standard EKG consists of, what eah lead represents, and correct placement of the electrodes.

The standard 12 lead EKG produces a picture of the heart's electrical activity. This is accomplished by recordring the heart in 12 different views. This is accomplished by placing 10 electrodes. 6 on the chest 2 on the arms and 2 on the legs. The leads (long wires) attached to the EKG machine are connected to the electrodes. Once connected, the EKG machine will record the heart's electrical activity from 12 different angles.

Let's now explore correct placement of the electrodes and their representation.

Limb leads: Limb leads also referred as frontal leads and record in a vertical plane. These leads describe the principle behind Einthoven's triangle. Although, Einthoven's triangle is not used in modern day EKG, it can be useful to detect incorrect lead placement.

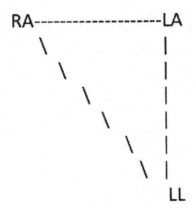

- Lead I (RA to LA)
- Lead II (RA to LL)
- Lead III (LA to LL)
- Augmented Vector Right (AVR)
- Augmented Vector Left (AVL)
- Augmented Vector Foot (AVF)

Electrode placement for the limb leads are as follows:

Right arm	(RA)	Between the right shoulder and right elbow.
Right Leg	(RL)	Between the right torso and above the right ankle.
Left arm	(LA)	Between the left shoulder and left elbow.
Left leg	(LL)	Between the left torso and the left ankle.

It should be noted that the right leg is neutral, meaning that the right leg is not recorded and is considered as a ground lead and aids in minimizing artifacts.

Precordial leads (Chest leads)- precordial leads also known as transverse leads. record the electrical activity in a horizontal plane. This is accomplised by attaching 6 electrodes on the patient's chest. The electrodes (V-leads) are are attached as follows.

- V1- Fourth intercostal (Between ribs), at the left border of the sternum.
- V2- Fourth intercostal space at the right border of the sternum.
- V3- Midway between V2 and V4.
- V4- Fifth intercostal space midclavicular line.
- V5- Anterior axillary (front of the armpit line), horizontal level as V4.
- V6- Mid-axillary (Mid-armpit line), horizontal level as V4 and V5.

Step-by-step Electrocardiogram procedure.

- Introduce yourself.
- Verify the patient by asking their name and date of birth.
- Explain the procedure.
- Ask the patient to remove clothing from the waist up and place the examination gown with the opening in front. You should exit the room while the patient is changing.
- If patient is wearing pants, role pant legs up half way. If the patient is wearing nylons ask the patient to remove the nylons. Electrodes cannot pick up electrical activity through nylons.
- Before beginning the procedure, ask the patient if they have any oils such as suntan lotion or baby oil on their skin. This can cause the electrodes to lose connection. Clean the areas where electrodes will be attached with alcohol.
- Explain to the patient that you will be placing electrodes on the arms, legs, and chest.
- Place the patient in the supine position (flat on back) with a pillow under their head for comport. If the supine poition is uncomfortable, place the patient in the semi-fowler's position (patient is in a 30 to 45 degree angle with a pillow under their head for comfort).
- Begin attaching electrodes on the patients limbs and chest. When placing the electrodes on the limbs, make sure they are placed on the fleshy part of the skin and not on bone.
- Type the patient's information into the EKG machine.
- Check the EKG machine is set at 25mm/sec (paper speed). This is viewable on the EKG machine.
- Check the EKG machine is set at 0.1 mV/mm. This records a 10mm standardization. Proper standardization confirms the height and width of the electrocardiogram is correct.
- Ask the patient to remain still until the procedure is complete
- Before removing electrodes, have the provider review the electrocardiogram. This is just in case the provider needs more recordings.

- Remove electrodes.
- Assist patient back in the sitting position. (Unless told differently by the provider).
- Thank patient and exit room.

Artifacts: Artifacts (interference) are not uncommon but can be reduced by following these steps.

- Before running the EKG machine, make sure the wires are not looping over each other. Wires looping over each other can affect the signal which can cause interference.
- Make sure the filter on the EKG machine is on. (The filter should never be turned off).
- Make sure the connectors are properly attached to the electrodes.
- Make sure chest hair is not affecting the placement of the electrode. This is done by moving the hair until you have some bare skin or shave the area where the electrodes will be attached. NOTE: Before shaving, you should explain to the and get permission from the patient so shave. It's also important that you follow the protocol of the facility. Some facilities do not allow shaving. Therefore, always check with the facility and the patient before you shave.
- Make sure there are no cracks in the wires. This should be done on a daily basis. This is usually completed first thing in the morning, before the day begins.
- Ask the patient to remove any jewelry they are wearing especially a watch with a second hand. The electrodes can sometimes pick up the movement of the second hand.
- You should place any jewelry the patient removes next to the patient. Never place jewelry in you lab coat.
- Aways use electrodes of of the same brand.
- Never attach electrodes on bone. Bone does not conduct electrity. The electrodes pick up electricity from the skin.

Additional note: If the patient has metal rods implanted this may cause interference. In this case complete the EKG and notify the provider.

Wave representation:

- **P wave:** The P wave is the first wave following the standardization. It represents the depolarization (contraction) of the atria.
- **QRS complex wave:** The QRS complex wave represents depolarization of the right and left ventricles. It is the most visable tracing.
- **T wave:** The T wave represents repolarization of the ventricles. (ventricles returning to their normal state).
- **ST Interval (segment):** The ST Segmant or interval represents the beginning of ventricular repolarization (the beginning of the ventricles returning to their normal state).
- **PR Interval:** The PR intrerval is the beginning of atrial depolarization, this is where the P wave appears until the beginning of the QRS complex wave. The beginning of ventricular depolarization.
- **U wave:** In a normal heartbeat the T wave represents ventricular repolarization. It is an extra wave following the T wave and sometimes can be missed. Although the U wave is not common, it appears when there is an electrolye (Potassium) imbalance.

To view a complete Elecrtrocardiogram, go to phlebotomy fundementals. com and click EKG.

Types of Elecrtrocardiograms: There are several types of ECG/EKG monitoring techniques. Some of the following tests require a cardiologist and sometimes a pulmonologist to be present. Let's begin.

Cardiopulmonary Excersise Test (CPET): Unlike the traditional stress test which assesses the heart by performing an EKG. The CPET is a complete cardiopulmonary tool which measures the amount of oxygen (O2) the patient's body is using and the amount of (CO2) the patient's body is producing. This test is peformed while the patient is riding a stationary bicycle. The following are some of the conditions the CPET can detect.

- Heart Failure- The heart is not pumping enough blood to the body's organs.
- Myocardial Ischemia-Due to blockage in either the small bloood vessels or large blood vessels blood flow is reduced to many parts of the heart.
- Pulmonary ventilation disorder- he lungs are unable to intake enough air to meet the body's needs. (ex: asthma, emphysema, COPD.
- Pulmonary circulation disorder- The body's inability to release oxygen from the lungs into the bloodstream. (ex: blood clot in the lungs).

Exercise Stress EKG: An exercise stress EKG also known as an exercise treadmill EKG is used to determine how well the heart responds when it's put under stress. It also is used to determine if the heart receives enough oxygen and proper blood flow. The test is just like performing a routine EKG. Sensors are attached to the skin. Buut instead of the patient being placed in the supine position, instead, the patient is walking slowy on a treadmill. During the test the speed and grade of the treadmill increase until the test is complete. The test can only be performed with the provider present.

Holtor Monitor: A holter monitor is a device used to track the heart rhythm and is usually ordered when the healthcare provider needs more information than what the traditional electrocardiogram can provide. The holter monitor is a small device and is worn for one to to days and records the heart rhythm for 24 to 48 hours. The patient may be asked to wear a holter for some of the following reasons.

- To detect arrhythmias that the traditional electrocardiogram may not detect.

- To determne if the heart medication is working.
- To detrmine if the heart is receiving enough oxygen.
- To determine why the patient has symptoms of dizziness or fainting (syncope) or the patient feels their heart is racing.

Chapter 11

Circulatory System/Vascular System

In this chapter we will be introducing the circulatory system and vascular system. The following will be covered.

- Cardiac cycle.
- Layers and struture of the heart.
- Types of blood vessels and their structure.
- Diagnostic tests of the circulatory system.
- Signs and symptoms of a heart attack.
- Disorders of the heart.
- Vascular system

The heart is a muscle which pumps oxygenated blood and nutrients to the blood vessels and body tissues. It is located in the thoracic cavity between the lungs. The tip of the of the heart called the apex faces downward toward the left of the body. The heart has four chambers. The top two chambers are called atria and the bottom two are called ventricles. The heart is also divided into left and right by the septum which is made up of cartilage. Between each atria and ventricle are valves. Valves allow blood to flow in one direction to prevent back flow. The heart is also surrounded by a fluid filled sac called the pericardium. The fluid called pericardial fluid keeps the heart lubricated to prevent friction while the heart is beating. Let's now begin to look in detail the anatomy of the Heart.

The heart consists of three layers, the epicardium, myocardium, and endocardium.

- **Epicardium:** The epicardium is a layer of muscle which covers the external surface of the heart. It is also fused with the myocardium and is also in contact with the pericardium
- **Myocardium:** The myocardium is the muscle layer of the heart. It aids in contraction and relaxation of the heart walls.
- Endocardium: The endocardium is the inner layer of the heart. It is made up of tissue which lines the chambers of the heart. The endocardium also protects the valves and the hearts chambers.

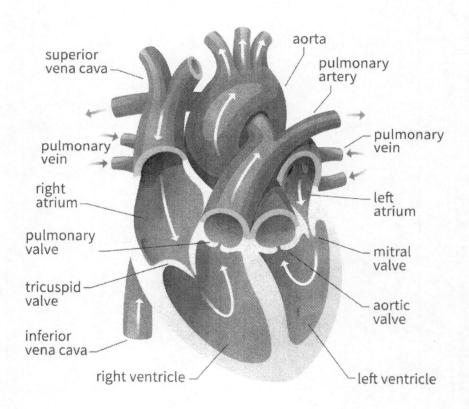

superior
vena cava

aorta

pulmonary
artery

pulmonary
vein

pulmonary
vein

right
atrium

left
atrium

pulmonary
valve

mitral
valve

tricuspid
valve

aortic
valve

inferior
vena cava

right ventricle

left ventricle

Valves of the heart: The purpse of the valves is to prevent back flow. They also reduce forward flow of blood. Should any of the valves not function correctly, the blood can back up and cause overflow of blood in th chamber which can put pressure on the heart causing the heart to work harder. Let's now examine each valve.

- **Tricuspid Valve:** This valve is located between the right atrium and right ventricle. It has three leaflets and its purpose is to prevent back flow of blood into the right atrium. If the valve does not close tightly, blood will back flow. This is called tricuspid valve regurgitation.

- **Mitral Valve:** This valve aslo known as the bicuspid vave is located between the left atrium and left ventricle. It has two leafs and it too prevents back flow of blood into the left atrium. If the valve does not close tightly, blood will back flow. This is called mitral valve regugitation which can put pressure on the left atrium and ultimately put pressure on the pulmonary veins, the veins which lead blood from the lungs to the heart.

- **Aortic Valve:** This valve is a semilunar valve and is between the left ventricle and the aorta. If the valve does not close tightly some of the blood which is oxygenated will back flow (regugitate) back into the left ventricle. This can cause the heart to work harder which can lead to hypertrophy (thickening of the heart muscle) making the heart less effective which ultimately can lead to heart failure.

- **Pulmonary Valve:** This valve also known as pulmonic valve has three leaflets and is located between the right ventricle and the pulmonary artery. If the valve fails to close tightly the blood will back flow to the right ventricle preventing the blood entering the lungs for oxygen. This condition is called pulmonary regurgitation.

Blood Vessels of the heart: There are five types of blood vessels and they vary in size. The vessels have three layers with the layers being thicker in arteries because that arteries expand and contract. Let's now look at types of vessels beginning with the layers.

- **Tunica Adventitia:** This layer known as tunica externa comes from the latin term for outer layer. It is made up of connctive tissue and as mentioned previously mentioned this layer is thicker in arteries. This is because arteries expand and contract.

- **Tunica Media:** This layer is the middle layer and is made up of smooth muscle cells and elastic fibers. The term tunica media is latin for middle layer.

- **Tunica intimia:** This layer is the inner most layer and is made up of endothelial cells and is covered by elastic tissue. The term tunica intimia is latin for inner layer.

- **Arteries:** Arteries carry oxygenated blood to the from the heart to the tissues organs of the body with one exception and that is the pulmonary artery. The pulmonary artery is carrying deoxygenated blood leading from the right ventricle to the lungs for oxygenation before it is returned to the left side of the heart.

- **Veins:** Veins return deoxygenated (poor oxygen) blood back to the heart with one exception, and that is the pulmonary vein which carries oxygenated blood from th lungs back to left side of the heart. Unlike arteries which pump blood throughout the body, veins work against gravity to bring blood back to the heart with thee assistance of skeletal muscles which contract, helping the blood flow back to the heart.

- **Arteriloes:** Arterioles branch out from the arteries and are part of the sympathetic nervous system (a part of the autonomic nervous system) and the purpose is to constrict, dilate, and regulate blood flow.

- **Venules:** Venules are small vessles which branch out from the veins ans allow deoxygenated blood to return to the veins via capillaries (microscop vessels).

- **Capillaries:** Capillaries are microscopic vessels which are about one cell thick and carry oxygenated blood along with nutrients to the tissues in the body; including, collecting carbon dioxide (CO_2), wast products, and fluids, and returning them to the veins.

Let's now follow the steps of blood flow through the heart:

- Superior Vena Cava
- Inferior Vena Cava
- Right Atrium
- Tricuspid Valve
- Right Ventricle
- Pulmonic valve
- Pulmonary Artery
- Pulmonary Vein
- Left Atrium
- Mitral Valve
- Left Ventricle
- Aortic Valve
- Aorta

Blood is then carried from the aorta through the body. (It should also be noted that once blood exits the pulmonary artery, blood enters the lungs for oxygenation and removal of carbon dioxide through the alveoli which are microscopic pouches before returning to the heart via the pulmonary vein).

Let's now begin exploring some of the common blood tests performed to aid in the detection of heart disease. Let's begin:

- **Cholesterol:** This test measures the amount of lipids (fat in the blood). It is a marker of risk factor of a heart attack (myocardial infarction), stroke or other vascular disease. A lipid panel includes; LDL, HDL, total cholesterol, and triglycerides. The most commonly used tube is a serum separator tube (SST). For an accurate LDL and triglyceride level, the patient should fast for 8-12 hours prior to the test.

Low Density Lipoprotein (LDL): also referred to (bad) cholesterol because too much can cause atherosclerosis (Build up of plaque in the arteries) which can reduce blood flow. Let's now look at LDL levels, catagories, and risk factors.

LDL Levels:

- Best: Less than 100mg/dL
- Target: 100-129 mg/dL
- Borderline High: 130-159mg/dL
- High: 160-189mg/dL
- Very High: 190+

Risk factors which can affect cardiac risk:

- High Blood Pressure (hypertension): in the past was 140/90. However, the American Heart Association has recently changed the the guideline from 140/90 to 130/80.
- Cigarette smoking
- HDL lower than 40mg/dL in men and less than 50mg/dl in women
- Family history
- Age (for men 45 years or older and women 55 years and older)

High Density Lipoprotein (HDL): Also referred to as (good) cholesterol because it aids in the removal of cholesterol from the arteries.

The HDL levels and catagories are as follows:

- Less than 40mg/dL: Risk factor for heart disease because the level of HDL is not high enough to fight the bad cholesterol LDL.
- 40-59 mg/dL: Levels are better but can be higher.
- 60 mg/dL and higher: This level is considered to be protective against heart disease.

Total Cholesterol: This is the total amount of cholesterol in the blood. This • includes LDL and HDL. The levels and catagories of total cholesterol for adults is as follows.

- Good: 200 mg/dL or less
- Borderline high: 200-239 mg/dL
- High: 240 mg/dl and higher

Triglycerides: This is a type of fat that is stored in the body and is used for energy. However, too much can raise the risk of heart disease. The levels and catagories of triglycerides is as follows.

- Normal: Less than 150 mg/dL
- Borderline High: 150-199 mg/dL
- High: 200-499 mg/dL

CRP (C reactive protein): C - reactive protein is produced by the liver in response to inflammation. The levels of CRP rise in various conditions such as possible inflammation of the arteries of the heart which, can be an indication of a high risk of a heart attack or stroke. The levels and catagories of CRP is as follows:

< 1.0 mg/L (low risk of cardiovascular disease)

1.0-3.0 mg/L (Averge risk of cardiovascular disease)

> 3.0 mg/L (high risk of cardiovascular disease)

Some conditions that could elevate the CRP:

- Heart Attack
- Vasculitis
- Lupus
- Rheumatoid Arthritis
- Burns
- Pneumonia
- Turbuculosis
- Trauma
- Inflammatory Bowel Disease
- Diabetes
- Obesity
- Certain cancers; such as colorectal cancer and lung cancer

The tube used to collect a CRP is an SST tube (serum separtor tube).

Potassium (K): potassium is an electrolyte and helps the muscles to contract and keeps the heartbeat regular. Low potassium in the blood is called hypokalemia. Too much potassium in the blood is called hyperkalemia. The tube used to collect potassium is an SST tube.

Creatnine Kinase (CK): Creatnine Kinase is an enzyme which the muscle cells of the body need in order to function properly. The levels of CK can rise after a heart attack, strenuous exercise, some medications and high intake of alcohol. The tube used to collect a CK is an SST tube.

Creatine Phosphokinase (CPK): CPK often rises and rushes to the bloodstream when there has been a significant of stress or injury to the heart muscle or brain. The tube used to collect a CPK is an SST tube.

Now that we have explored some of the diagnostic tests performed to aid in detecting possible heart disease, let's now explore in detail some of the following cardiac disorders.

- Heart Attack (Myocardial Infarction)
- Coronary Artery Disease (CAD)
- Abnormal Heart Rhythm (Arrhythmia)
- Heart Failure
- Heart Muscle Disease (Cardiomyopathy)

Heart Attack (Myocardial Infarction):

Every year, approximately 735,000 people in the United States suffer a heart attack (myocardial infarction) and they can come on sudden or in many cases, will come on slow usually with mild pain and discomfort. Should the patient complain of the following symptoms, immediately stop what your are doing and call 911 and inform the healh care provider. In many institutions, a code is called. Under no circumstances should you ever leave the patient unattended. Always remain witn the patient until responders arrive.

- **Chest Discomfort:** In many cases, chest discomfort will appear and sometimes can last for a few minutes and disappear and then return. The patient may tell you that they feel chest pain, squeezing pressure. If possible, ask the patient how long they have been experiencing the symptoms. It is very helpful to the healthcare provider and responders.

- **Shortness of Breath (SOB):** Shortness of breath can occur whether or not the patient is experiencing a heart attack. Ask the patient how long they have been experiencing shortness of breath and notify the provider.
- Discomfort in the upper body: Along with chest discomfort and pain, the patient may also experience discomfort in the jaw, one or both arms, the back, neck, and stomach.

It should also be noted that other symptoms such as breaking out in a cold sweat, nausea or lightheadedness can occur.

Symptoms also vary between men and women for instance, women, most often experience shortness of breath, nausea, vomiting back or jaw pain.

Coronary Artery Disease (CAD)/
Coronary Heart Disease (CAD):

Coronary artery disease occurs when plaque begins building up against the walls of the coronary artery which results in poor blood supply to the heart's muscle (myocardium). This is also known as ischemia and it can be chronic or acute. In fact, coronary artery disease leads to coronary heart disease and can be prevented by living a healthy lifetyle such as a diet low in saturated fats, cholesterol, optimally treating high blood pressure (hypertension), maintaining a normal body weight and exercising.

(It should also be noted, that coronary artery disease begins in childhood years).

Risk factors include:

- Smoking
- Diabetes
- Obesity
- High LDL cholesterol
- Low HDL cholesterol
- High Blood Pressure
- Post menopausal women

Risk factors that can't be changed:

- Heredity- Family history of heart disease.
- Race- African americans, have a higher risk of heart disease.
- Gender- Men have a great risk of heart attack than women.
- Age- People who die from coronary heart disease are generally 65 or older.

Abnormal heart rhythm (Arrhythmia): An arrhythmia is when the heart beats too fast, too slow, or the beats are irregular. It is for this reason, when you are feeling a pulse, it is extremely important to pay close attention to each beat and count the number of skip beats. For instance, while taking the pulse you counted 84 beats in one minute, but, you also counted 5 skipped beats. This should be reported and recorded as P 84 with 5 skipped beats.

Let's now explore some types of arrhythmias.

- **Bradycardia:** When the heart rate is less than 60 beats per minute (BPM), the patient is said to have bradycardia. Bradycardia occurs when the signals from the atria and the ventricles become disrupted. However, not all patients who have a heart rate of less than 60 beats per minute have a heart problem. For instance, people who are in excellent physical condition may have slower heart rates.

- **Tachycardia:** When the resting heart rate is greater than 100 beats per minute (BPM) the patient is said to have tachycardia. There are several types of tachycardia. Let's explore a couple of them.

1. **Ventricular tachycardia:** Is a condition where the ventricles receive abnormal electrical from the atria, and because, the ventricles are beating so fast they do not have time to fill correctly, which can lead to the heart not being able to pump enough blood to the lungs and body. Ventricular tachycardia (VT) can in some cases cause the heart to stop (sudden cardiac arrest). Ventricular tachycardia can cause symptoms (Sx) of lightheadedness, palpitations, dizziness, and in some cases the patient may lose consciousness.

2. **Sinus Tachycardia:** Sinus tachycardia occurs often when the body's demand for oxygenated blood increases, such as in stress, dehydration, exercise or illness.

Angine pectoris: Angina, is caused by lack of blood flow to the heart due to coronary artery disease. Symptoms of angina include:

- Chest discomfort
- Pain in the arms, neck, shoulder, jaw, or back along with chest pain.
- Nausea/vomiting
- Sweating
- Shortness of breath (SOB)

Vascular System: The vascular system is made up of vessels that carry blood. The lymph system returns fluid or lymph.atic fluid. Lymphatic fluid is a colorless, clear fluid which is carried through the lymph channels and helps to maintain and protect the fluid of the body by filtering and expelling lymph away from the body,

As previously mentioned, the circulatory system is comprised of vessels which carry blood throughout the body by the pumping action of the heart. The heart begins to pump oxygenated blood through the arteries. Arteries branch out into smaller vessels called arterioles which send oxygen and nutrients to the bodies tissues, cells, and organs. Blood then flows into microscopic vessels called capillaries. Capillaries send oxygen and nutrients to the cells. The vascular system has additional functions that are important to other body systems. Let's look into each system.

- **Digestive system:** Upon digestion, blood flow through capillaries which pick up nutrients such as, glucose, vitamins, and minerals. The nutrients are delivered to body's tissues by the blood.
- **Respiratory system:** Blood flows through the capillaries into the lungs where carbon dioxide is expelled from the body through the lungs, and oxygen is taken to the body's tissues through the blood.

- **Kidneys/Urinary system:** Waste material is filtered out from the blood as it flows through the kidneys. Waste is expelled from the body in the form of urine.
- **Temperature Control:** The body's temperature is regulated by the flow of blood through different parts of the body. It should also be noted that the body's tissues produce heat by breaking down nutrients for energy, production of new tissue and expelling waste.

Let's now look at some disorders of the vascular system including some diagnostic tests used to diagnose these disorders.

- **Arteriosclerosis:** Arteriosclerosis is the hardening of the arteries and over time, blood flow to the body's organs and tissues can become restricted. The following are some factors which can contribute.
  - High blood pressure (hypertension)
  - High cholesterol (hypercholesterolemis)
  - Obesity
  - Smoking
  - Diabetes

- **Atherosclerosis:** Atherosclerosis is the plaque bulidup in the lining of the arteries. The buildup is from fatty substances such as cholesterol, calcium, fibrin, and waste products. The thickening of plaque buildup causes the narrowing of the arteries which can decrease or completely block the flow of blood the body's organs, tissues, and structures. It should be noted that, atherosclerosis can begin as early as childhood.
- **Inflammation:** Inflammation such as vasculitis (inflammation of the blood vessels) can lead to the narrowing and blockage of the blood vessels.
- **Blood clots:** A tiny mass (embolus) or blood clot (thrombus) moving through the blood stream can block a blood vessel.

- **Aneurysm:** An aneurysm, also referred as the silent killer is when the wall of a blood vessel, most often an artery weakens causing the vessel to balloon out. Aneurysms, often have no symptoms (Sx) and can develop over years. Aneurysms can expand and rupture. The following sympoms can include:
  - Dizziness/Vertigo
  - Nausea and Vomiting
  - Clammy skin
  - Pain
  - Rapid Heart Rate
  - Low blood pressure
  - Severe or worst ever headache
  - Shock

Embolism: An embolism is the blockage of material (embolus) in the blood vessel. An embolus can be in the form of a blood clot (thrombus), fat globule

Risk Factors can include:

- Family history
- High Blood Pressure (hypertension)
- High Cholesterol (Hypercholesterolemia)
- Smoking

- **Phlebitis:** Phlebitis is the inflammation of a vein and can occur in both the superficial veins (veins on the skin surface) or deep veins also known as deep vein thrombophlebitis (DVT). Let's explore each one in detail.
- Superficial phlebitis- Superficial phlebitis can occur from the following.

  - Probing the vein- Probing a vein with the needle inserted to obtain blood can cause trauma to the vein resulting in phlebitis.

- Multiple needle punctures- Multiple needle punctures cause trauma to the vein which can result in phlebitis.
- Intravenous IV can cause irritation to a vein.
- Blood clot- Phlebitis can also be caused by blood clot (thrombus).
- Medications- Some medicatons administered through the veins can cause the vein becoming irritated.

- **Deep Vein Thrombophlebitis (DVT):** Deep vein thrombosis is blood clot that has formed in one of the deep veins usually in the legs. DVT can cause swelling (edema) and leg pain. DVT is a serious condition because if one or more of the blood clots break away, they can travel through the bloodstream and into the lungs preventing blood flow. This is know an a pulmonary embolism. It is also important to know that deep vein thrombisis can occur without symptoms.

Let's now examine some of the risk factors of deep vein thrombosis.

- Smoking- Smoking increases the risk of DVT
- Sitting for long periods of time- Lack of leg movement for long periods of time can cause the calf muscles to not contract causing clots to form in the legs.
- Family history (Hx) of DVT- Family history increases the risk of developing DVT.
- Age- Patients older than 60 have a greater risk of developing DVT.
- Heart Failure- Patients with heart failure, have a greater risk of developing DVT and pulmonary embolism because heart and lung function are limited.
- Overweight/Obesity- Patients who are overweight or obese are at risk of developing DVT because, pressure on the veins in the pelvis and legs become increased.
- Pregnancy- During pregnancy, the risk factor of pressure in the veins of the pelvis and legs increases. The risk factor for DVT can continue for up to six weeks after delivery.

- Inflammatory bowel disease- Bowel disease such as Ulcerative Colitis or Crohn's disease increase the risk of developing DVT.

- **Varicose veins:** Varicose veins are enlarged veins caused by weakened valves and veins of the legs. Once the veins become weakened, they become enlarged and begin to twist. For some patients, varicose veins or spider veins may simply be cosmetic. However, for some patients, varicose veins can be painful and lead to serous health problems. Let's now explore some causes associated with varicose veins

Causes of vericose veins:

- **Pregnancy:** Pregnancy can increase the chances of developing varicose veins because during the pregnancy, the volume of blood increases but at the same time blood flow decreases from the legs to the pelvis in order to support the fetus. The change of blood flow can cause the veins of the legs to become enlarged. In most cases, after a few months after delivery, the vericose veins disappear without any form of medical treatment.
- **Age:** As person ages, the valves in the veins weaken, causing the blood which should be returning to the heart to backflow causing blood to build up in the veins causing the veins to enlarge and become varicose.
- **Obesity:** Obesity can put additional pressure on the legs veins and valves and over time the buildup of pressure causes the veins to enlarge and become vericose.

Common diagnostic test of the vascular system:

- **Lipoprotein:** Lipoprotein transports cholesterol and triglycerides in the blood stream. normal lipoprotein levels are less than 30 mg/dl. Lipoprotein levels greater than 30 mg/dl may be an indication of increased risk of heart attack or stroke. The tube uses to collect a lipoprotein is an Serum Separator Tube (SST).

- **Prothrombin Time (PT/INR):** A prothrombin time (PT) and international normalized ration (INR) is a test to determine how long it takes for the blood to clot. The normal range for PT/INR in patients not taking blood thinners such as coumadin or warfarin is- PT 11 to 13.5 seconds and INR 0.8 to .1.1. The tube used for a PT/INR is a light blue top tube which contains the anticoagulant sodium citrate. The tube must be full and inverted at least six times to ensure proper mixing of the anticoagulant with the blood. To prevent contamination of excess tissue in the blood, draw a discard tube such as a red top or SST tube prior to collecting the PT/INR.

- **Partial Thromboplastin Time (PTT)/ Activated Patrial Thromboplastin Time (APTT):** Both partial thromboplastin time and activated partial thromboplastin time measure blood coagulation (clotting). The only difference is that an APTT is a much more sensitive test and is used for patients on heparin therapy. The range for PTT is 60-70 seconds. The range for APPT is 30-40 seconds. The tube used for a PTT or APTT is a light blue top tube which contains the anticoagulant sodium citrate. The tube must be full and inverted six times to ensure proper mixing of the anticoagulant and blood. To prevent contamination of excess tissue in the blood, draw a discard tube such as a red top tube or SST tube prior to collecting a PTT or APTT.

- **Triglycerides:** Triglycerides are fat in the blood and give energy to the body. High levels of triglycerides can lead to heart disease. Triglyceride levels are as follows. Normal – less than 150 mg/dl, Borderline- 150-199 mg/dl, High- 200-499mg/dl. The tube used to collect triglyceride is a serum separator tube (SST). For optimal results, the patient should fast 8-12 hours prior to the test.

Chapter 12

Respiratory System

In this chapter, we will be covering in detail the respiratory system. The following will be covered.

- Function of the respiratory system
- Structure of the respiratory system
- Disorders of the respiratory system
- Common Diagnostic tests of the respiratory system

Function of the respiratory system: Although the primary function of the respiratory system is the exchange of oxygen (O2) and carbon dioxide (CO2), the respiratory system has five functions. Let's explore each function in detail. Let's begin.

- Inhalation and Exhalation- As air is inhaled through the nasal and oral cavity it passes through the pharynx (throat), larynx (voicebox), trachea (windpipe) and into the lungs. Once the process of gas exchanges has occurred in the lungs, air is then exhaled through the same path as inhalation.
- External respiration- Inside the lungs, there are millions of microscopic sacs called alveoli. It is here where oxygen from inhaled air is circulated from the alveoli into the capillaries and become fixed to hemoglobin in the red blood cells, and

pumped through the red blood cells (erythrocytes) in the bloodstream. At the same time carbon dioxide is circulated from the capillaries into the alveoli and is exhaled. This process is called external respiration.

- Internal Respiration- Internal respiration is the process of which the red blood cells, deliver oxygen which has been absorbed from the

HUMAN RESPIRATORY SYSTEM

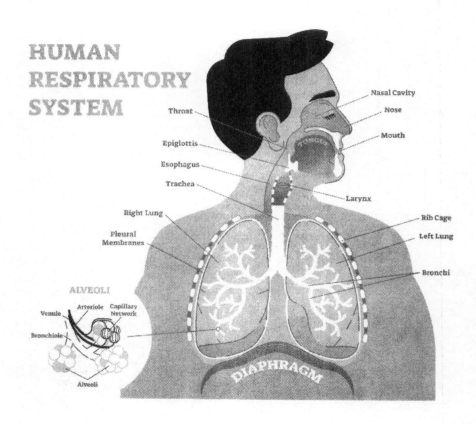

lungs through the blood vessels of the body. The oxygenated blood, travels through the microscopic capillaries where the red blood cells will release oxygen to the body's tissues. At the same time, carbon dioxide is released from the tissues and returned to the red blood cells and plasma. Deoxygenated blood along carbon dioxide return back to the lungs to be expelled.

- **Vibration of the vocal cords**- During the process of exhalation, air in the lungs passes through the larynx (voice box) where muscles in the larynx move cartilages. The cartilages push the vocal cords together. Air then passes between the cords which make them vibrate, creating sound.
- **Olfactory (sense of smelling)**- When air enters the nasal cavity, chemicals in the air fasten and initiate the receptors of the nervous system. These receptors are called cilia (hair like structures). These receptors move the signals to the brain where neurons send the signals to the etmoid bone to the olfactory bulbs. Finally, the signals from the olfactory bulbs move along the cranial nerve to the olfactory area of the cerbral cortex where sense of smell occurs.
- **Structures of the respiatory system**- The respiatory system is made up of the following structures. The nose, mouth, pharynx, larynx, trachea, bronchi, bronchioles, alveoli, lungs, and muscles of the respiratory system. Let's now look into each structure and their fuction in detail. Let's begin.
- **Nose**- The nose is the entry way to the respiratory tract. Along with providing air to the respiratory tract, it filters, moistens, and warms the air during inhalation. Inside the nose ther is a mucous membrane. The membrane is moist and contains hairlike structures called cilia and it's function is to remove foreign debris such as dust. The nose is also, seperated into right and left by a wall of cartilage called the septum. It also consists the olfactory organ which contains receptors of sense and smell.
- **Mouth**- The mouth, also referred to the oral or buccal cavity is where food and air enter. It's primary role however is the initial

intake of food and digestion. We will cover the mouth in more detail when we cover the digestive system.

- **Pharynx (Throat)**- The pharynx, which is connected to the larynx, is the passageway for both food and air. During swallowing, a thin layer of cartilage called the epiglottis, blocks the opening to the larynx, allowing food to go down the esophagus which leads to the stomach.

- **Larynx (voicebox)**- The larynx s about 2 inches in length and is located between the pharynx and trachea. The larynx, aids in breathing, swallowing, and speaking. The outer wall of the cartilage which forms in the front of the neck and is referred as the Adams apple.

- **Trachea (Windpipe)**- The trachea, also known as the wind pipe is 4 inches long and lies behind the larynx and continues down behind the sternum (breastbone). The trachea divides into two smaller branches called bronchi. There is one bronchus for each lung. The function of the trachea is to provide air to and from the lungs.

- Bronchi- The primary function of the bronchi is to deliver oxygen to the lungs during inhalation and to expel carbon dioxide through the trachea during exhalation. It should be noted, bronchi is plural for bronchus.

- **Bronchioles**- Each bronchus, divides into smalller branches called bronchioles. The main function of the bronchioles is to deliver air into each alveolus. Each lung contains approximately 30,000 bronchioles and are approximately 1mm in diameter.

- **Alveoli**- Bronchioles, later divide into microscopic sacs called alveoli. The primary function of the alveoli is the exchange of oxygen and carbon dioxide. When inhaled oxygen reaches the alveoli, it moves the oxygen to the blood in the capillaries, meanwhile, carbon dioxide, moves from the blood in each alveoli and is exhaled. Depending on the size of the lung, the number of alveoli can be anywhre from 300 million to over 700 million alveoli.

- **Lungs**- The lungs are spongy and are located on either side of the chest also known as the thorax. A thin layer of tissue called the pleura covers each lung. Each lung also contains a thin layer of fluid called plural fluid. The fluid lubricates the lungs which allows them to expand and contract easily.
- Muscles of the respiratory system- The main muscle of the respiratory system is the diaphragm. The diaphragm, is a dome-shaped muscle that separates the abdominal cavity from the thoracic cavity. During inhalation the diaphragm contracts allowing the lungs to expand. Meanwhile, the intercostal muscles between the ribs move upward and outward during inhalation. During exhalation, the diaphragm relaxes and moves back up and the chest walls push the air out of the lungs.

Now that we have examined the function and structures of the respiratory system, lets now look at some disorders of the respiratory system. Let's begin.

Disorders of the respiratory system:

- Apnea (Sleep Apnea)- Sleep apnea is a serous breathing disorder where breathing constantly stops and starts. Some of the most common symptoms of sleep apnea are as follows:
  - Loud snoring
  - Morning headache
  - awakening with a dry mouth or sore throat
  - Attention difficulties
  - Irritability

- **Asthma**- Asthma is a controllable, non-curable condition where the airways narrow and swell making breathing difficult. Asthma can be caused by irritants that cause allergies (Allergens) or genetic factors (inherited). It should be noted that it is unclear why some people develop asthma while others do not. Let's now look into some causes and symptoms of asthma.

Causes:

- Respiratory infections, such as a cold
- Exposure to cold air
- Airborne substances, such as pet dander, dust mites, pollen, mold, cockroach waste.
- Medications, such as asprin, ibuprofen
- Air pollutants, such as smoke

Symptoms:

- Shortness of Breath (SOB)
- Caughing or Wheezing
- Whistling or wheezing during exhalation (common in children)
- Chest tightness

Bronchitis- Bronchitis is the inflammation of the mucous membrane of the bronchial tubes. Bronchitismay be either acute (sudden onset) or chronic (long term or constantly reaccuring). Let's now look at some causes and symptoms of bronchitis.

Causes:

Acute Bronchitis- Acute bronchitis can be caused by viruses, such as a cold or influenza.

Chronic Bronchitis- Cigarette smoke is the most common cause of bronchitis. However, otheer causes of chronic bronchitis are; dust, air pollution, toxic gases.

Symptoms: Symptoms for acute or chronic bronchitis include:

- Non-productive
- Productive cough (sputum). Sputum (phlegm) can be clear, yellow, or green. Although rare, some blood my be present.
- Shortness of breath

- Chest discomfort
- fatigue
- fever (slight) or chills

Cystic Fibrosis- (CF) Cystic fibrosis is a progressive hereditary disease that affects the exocrine glands (glands that produce and secrete sustances such as salivary glands, sweat glands, and mammary glands.

Cystic fibrosis also causes damage to the lungs and other body organs. And because screening and treatments (Tx) have improved patients are living a better quality of life with some patients living into their 40's and 50's. Let's now look at some of the causes and symptoms of cystic fibrosis.

Causes: The cause of cystic fibrosis is the mutation (defect) in a gene that changes a protein which regulates the movement of salt in and out of the cells.

Symptoms (Respiratory system)

- Wheezing
- Persistant productive cough with thick sputum (phlegm/Musus)
- Continuous lung infectons
- Breathlessness

Symptoms (Digestive system)

- Intestininal blockage
- Severe constipation
- Unpleasent-smell, greasy stool
- Poor weight gain

Dyspnea (difficulty breathing or shortness of breath)- Dyspnea can be acute (comes on suddenly) or chronic (long lasting). Let's now explore some of the causes. Let's begin.

Causes (Acute)

- Asthma
- Carbon monoxide poisoning
- Heart attack (myocardial Infarction)
- Low blood pressure (Hypotension)
- Pneumonia
- Pulmonary embolism (Blood clot in an artery in the lung)
- Upper airway obstruction

Causes (Chronic)

- Asthma
- COPD (Chronic Obstructive Pulmonary Disease)
- Obesity
- Lung Cancer
- Pleurisy (Inflammation of the pleural membrane surrounding the lungs)
- Pulmonary Edema (Excessive fluid build-up in the lungs)
- Tuberculosis

Emphysema- Emphysema is a progressive lung disease where the alveoli (air sac in the lungs) are damaged, reducing the amount of oxygen to enter the bloodstream. In many cases, patients with emphysema, also have chronic bronchitis. Let's now look at some causes of emphysema.

Causes:

- Air pollutants
- Chemical fumes
- Tobacco (including exposure to second hand smoke)

Hypoxia/Hypoxemia- Hypoxia is a condition where there is an insufficient amount of oxygen reaching the body's tissues. Hypoxemia, is the insufficient amount of oxygen to the bloodstream. Both hypoxia and hypoxemia may be acute or chronic. Let's look at some causes and symptoms.

Causes:

- Chronic Obtructive Pulmonary Disease (COPD)
- Anemia
- Cyanide poisoning

Symptoms:

- Cough
- Rapid heart rate
- Rapid breathing
- Shortness of Breath
- Wheezing

Pleurisy- Pleurisy is the inflammation of the pleura (the tissue layers of the lungs). Lets now look at some causes and symptoms of pleurisy.

Causes:

- Cancer
- Congestive Heart Failure (CHF)
- Pulmonary embolism (Blood clot in an artery of the lungs)
- Tuberculosis (TB)

Symptoms:

- Chest pain
- Shortness of breath

Pneumonia- Pneumonia is an infection which inflames the air sacs of one or both lungs. The air sacs can also fill up with fluid which causes coughing up phlegm (sputum), difficulty breathing, fever, and chills. Let's now look at some causes and symptoms of pneumonia.

Causes: There are many germs tht can cause pneumonia and are classified by the location where the germ was aquired. Let's look at each location in detail.

Community-aquired pneumonia- This is the most common type of pneumonia and is aquired outside the healthcare facility and can be caused by:

- **Bacterial pneumonia**- This type of pneumonia is common and typically after a cold or flu. This type of pneumonia is caused by the bacteria streptococcus pneumoniae.
- **Fungi**- This type of pneumonia occurs mostly in patients with weakened immune systems or chronic health issues. This type of pneumonia is caused by fungi found in soil, or bird droppings.
- Viruses- Viral pneumonia can be caused by a cold or flu. In most cases, viral pneumonia is mild but can become serious.

Hospital- aquired pneumonia- This type of pneumonia occurs in patients who are hospitalized for other illnessess, and can be serious because certain types of bacteria can be antibiotic resistant.

Healthcare-aquired pneumonia- This type of pneumoni affects patients lining in long term care facilities or out patient clinics.

Aspiration pneumonia- This type of pneumonia occurs when drinks, food, or vomit are inhaled into the lungs. Aspiration pneumonia generally occurs with excessive use of alcohol, drugs or brain injury.

Symptoms:

- Chest pain (during breathing or coughing)
- Fatigue
- Fever
- Nausea or vomiting
- Productive cough
- Shortness of breath

Pulmonary edema- Pulmonary edema is the accumulation of fluid in the air sacs of the lungs, making breathing difficult. Symptoms of pulmonary edema can develop suddenly (acute) or can be long term (chronic). Let's explore some of the symptoms.

Acute pulmonary edema:

- Wheezing
- Feeling of suffocating
- Dyspnea (difficulty breathing), worsens when lying down
- Productive cough with frothy sputum and in some cases, blood could be present.
- Rapid or irregular heart rhythm
- patients with heart disease may develop pulmonary edema

Chronic pulmonary edema:

- Wheezing
- Swellling in lower extemities
- Fatigue
- Dyspnea (difficulty breathing) when lying down or with exertion

Tuberculosis (TB)- Tuberculosis is an infectious disease caused by the mycobacterium tuberculosis bacterium. It is spread into the air through tiny droplets when a person coughs or sneezes. Tuberculosis, generally affects the lungs, however, tuberculosis can affect other parts of the body such as the brain, spine, and kidneys.

It should be noted, that patients who are coughing, should be asked to wear a face maks to prevent the spread of droplets entering the air.

Symptoms of active TB include:

- Coughs lasting more than three weeks
- Chest pain, or pain when breathing or coughing
- Coughing up blood

- Fatigue
- Fever
- chills
- Night sweats
- Loss of appetite

Upper Resperatory Infection (URI)- An upper respiratory infection (URI) or also known as the common cold ae contracted when a person is in contact with an airborne virus usually from droplets for sneezing or coughing. Upper respiratory infections are contagious and spread from person to person. The virus can also be contracted from poor hand washing. The particles then pass from one person to another. People who are at a greater risk of contracting a URI are people with a poor immune system. Let's now look at some symptoms of a URI.

Symptoms:

- Sneezing
- Runny nose
- Sore throat
- Cough
- Headache
- Nasal and sinus blockage

Diagnostic tests:

- Alkaline phosphatase (ALP) Serum Separator Tube (SST)
- Arterial Blood Gas (ABG) Usually performed by IV nurse or provider
- Blood Cultures (BC) Arobic and anarobic vials
- Complete Blood Count (CBC) Lavender top tube
- Electolytes (Lavender top tube)
- Oximetry (oxineter used to test the amount of oxygn is in the blood)
- PPD/Mantoux/TB test (test used to screen for tuberculosis)

Chapter 13

The Nervous System

In This chapter, we will be introducing the nervous system. The following will be covered.

- Function of the nervous system
- Structure of the nervous system
- Disorders of the nervous system
- Common diagnostic tests of the nervous system

Function of the nervous system: The nervous system has three main functions. They are:

- Sensory nerves that take information from inside the body and the outside environment. The nerves, then carry all the information gathered to the central nervous system (CNS).
- Information gathered is sent to the central nervous system, where the information is processed and interpreted.
- Motor nerves send information form the central nervous system to the muscles and glands of the body.

Structures of the nervous system: The nervous system is made up of brain, spinal cord, and nerves. Together they all comminucate. For instance, the brain and spinal cord together make up the central nervous system (CNS). This is where the information is received, evaluated, and decisions are made. Another division of the nervous system is the peripheral nervous system (PNS). This is where the sensory nerves and sense organs control and monitor the conditions of the body, inside and out and information is then sent to the central nervous system. Let's now begin to break down the central nervous system beginning with neurons. Let's begin.

Human Brain *Diagram*

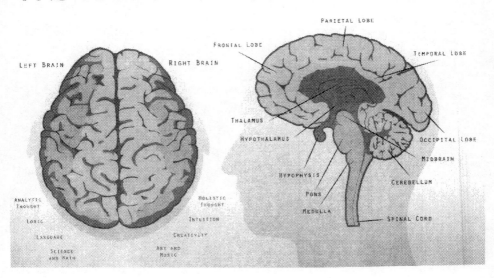

133

Neurons- Neurons, make up the nerves and brain. they communicate by sending electrochemical signals within the body. Unlike other cells within the body, neurons look different. First, there is a cell body. The cell body is the round part of the neuron that contains the nucleus, mitochondria, and many of the cellular organelles (specialized structures in a living cell). Next, there are tiny, tree like structures called dendrites. Dendrites, extend from the cell body which pick up stimuli from the enviroment and other neurons. Next are axons. Axons are the long slender part of a nerve cell that conducts electrical impulses away from the neuron's cell body. In essence, axons are the primary lines of the nervous system. Additionally, each neuron in the body is surrounded by neuroglia. Neuroglia, feed, protect, and insulate the neuron. protect, and insulate the neuron.

There are three classes of neurons they are afferent neurons, efferent neurons, and interneurons. Let's look at each one individually.

- **Afferent neurons-** Afferent or sensory neurons transmit signals to the central nervous system from receptors in the body.
- **Efferent neurons-** Efferent or motor neurons transmit signals from the central nervous system to the effectors in the body.
- **Interneurons-** Interneurons are complex networks within the central nervous system which put together the information received from the afferent neurons and direct the function of the body through the efferent neurons.

Brain- The brain, is located in the cranial cavity and weighs approximately 3 pounds and is made up of the cerebrum, cerebullum, and brain stem. The brain is divide into right and left hemispheres. The right side of the brain controls creativity, and, artistic musical skills. The left side of the brain controls comprehension, speech, arithmetic, and writing. It should also be noted, that the left side of the brain largely controls language, and hand use.

Layers of the brain and spinal cord- The brain and spinal cord are protected by three layers of tisse called the meninges. The layers are: dura mater, arachnoid, and pia mater. Let's explore each layer.

- **Dura mater**- The dura mater is a thick membrane that lines the inside of the skull. The term dura mater is latin for tough mother.
- **Arachnoid mater**- The arachnoid mater is made up of elastic tissue. It is a thin, web-like membrane that covers the entire brain. The space between the dura mater and arachnoid mater Is the subdural space.
- **Pia Mater**- The pia mater contains many blood vessels that stretch deep into the brain. Between the arachnoid and pia mater is the subarachnoid space. The subarachnoid space contains cerebral spinal fluid (CSF) which acts a cushion for the brain. The term pia mater is latin for soft mother.

Lobes of the brain- The brain is divided into four lobes: Frontal, temporal, parietal, and occipital. Let's now look into rhe function of each lobe.

Frontal lobe- The frontal lobe controls the following:

- Personality, behavior, and emotions
- Planning, problem solving, and judgement
- Speech (speaking and writing)
- Body movement (motor)
- Intelligence, self awareness, and concentration

Temporal lobe- The temporal lobe controls the following:

- Memory
- hearing
- understanding language
- organization and sequencing

Parietal lobe- The parietal lobe controls the following:

- Sense of touch, pain, and temperature
- Interprets signals from hearing, vision, sensory, memory, and motor, visual spatial perception.
- Interprets language and words

Occipital lobe- th occipital lobe controls the following:

- Interprets vision including; color, light, and movement

Deep inside the brain, there are deep structures, they are the hypothalamus, pituitary gland, pineal gland, and thalamus. Let's now into each deep structure of the brain.

- **Hypothalamus**- The hypothalamus is the main control center of the autonomic system. It controls thirst, hunger, sleep, andd sexual response. The hypothalamus also regulates blood pressure, body temperature, emotions, ans secretions of hormones.
- **Pituitary gland**- Referred to as the "master gland" the pituitary gland is located beneath the hypothalamus and is about the size of a pea. The pituitary gland secretes the hormones that control sexual development, aids in bone and muscle growth, and responds to stress.
- **Pineal gland**- The pineal gland secretes melatonin, and aids in the role of sexual development.
- **Thalamus**- The role of the thalamus is pain sensation, alertness, attention, and memory.

Spinal cord- Approx 18 inches in length, the spinal cord runs within a protective spinal canal from the brainstem to the first lumbar vertabra. The spinal nerves continue down to the tail bone and branch off to the legs and feet. The role of the spinal cord is to relay messages between the brain and the body.

Spinal nerves- There are 31 pairs of spinal nerves that branch off from the spinal cord. The spinal nerves carry messages back and forth between the body and spinal cord allowing control of sensation and movement. The spinal nerves are numbered according the location of the vertabra. They are as follows:

- Cervical spinal nerves C1-C8
- Thoracic spinal nerves T1-T12
- Lumbar spinal nerves L1-L5
- Sacral spinal nerves S1-S5
- The coccygeal nerve has one nerve

Cranial nerves- The brain communicates through the spinal cord and twelve pairs of cranial nerves. The cranial nerves which originate from the brainstem control hearing, facial expression, eye movement, taste, swallowing, movement of the face, neck, shoulder, and muscles of the tongue. The cranial nerves which originate from the cerebrum contol vision and sense of smell.

Peripheral nervous system (PNS)- The peripheral nervous system are all the nerves that lie outside of the central nervous system. The main role of the peripheral nervous system is connecting the central nervous system to the organs, limbs, and skin. The peripheral nervous system is divided into two parts. Each part is is critical in how the peripheral nervous system operates. The two parts are the somatic nervous system and the autonomic nervous system. Let's look at each part.

Somatic nervous system- The somatic nervous system transmits sensory information including involuntary movement. The somatic nervous system has to types of neruons, sensory and motor.

Sensory neurons- Sensory neurons transmit information from the nerves to the central nervous system. The information is then sent to the brain and spinal cord.

Motor neurons- Motor neurons, transmit information from the brain and spinal cord. The information is sent to muscle fibers throughout the body.

Autonomic nervous system- The autonomic nervous system controls the body's internal processes such as:

- Heart rate
- Breathing
- Blood pressure
- Metabolism
- Digestion
- Water and electolyte balance (such as sodium (NA+ or potassium K+)
- Body temperature
- Production of body fluids (such as saliva)
- Urination
- Defecation
- Sexual response

The autonomic nervous system also has two main divisions, the sympathetic and parasympathetic nervous system. Let's explore each one.

- **Sympathetic nervous system**- the sympathetic nervous system responds and prepares the body in stressful situations Iso known as fight or flight. For example, when a person is in a situation where they need too defend themselves, the sympathetic system increase heart rate. The increased heart rate causes the airways to dilate (widen). Muscles become strengthened, and stored energy in the body is released. At the same time, other body processes such as digestion are decreased.
- **Parasympathetic nervous system**- The parasympathetic nervous system restores and controls the body in normal situations such as it slows the heart rate and decreases heart rate including stimulization of the digestive tract.

Now that we have explored some of the functions and structures of the nervous system, let's now look at some disorders of the nervous system. Let's begin.

Alzheimer's disease- Alzheimer's disease is a progressive disease which ultimately destroys memory along with many other mental functions. Over time, patients with Alzheimer's disease will forget people in their lives along with dramatic personality changes. Let's look at the causes risk factors, and symptoms associated with Alzheimer's disease.

Causes- Although, the causes of Alzheimer's disease is not completely understood, scientists believe the cause of Alzheimer's disease is caused by the enviroment, lifestyle, genetics or a combination of all. What is know's that Alzheimer's disease destroys and kills brain cells. As more brain cells are destroyed, the disease leads to brain shrinkage.

Risk factors-

- **Family history**- It appears that patients have a higher risk of developing Alzheimer's if a parent or sibling (also known as first degree relative) has the disease. Although there have been many break throughs, there are many gene factors that cannot be conclusively comfirmed.
- **Age**- Developing Alzheimer's disease, greatly ingreases with age. Although Alzheimer's disiease is not a part of the aging prosess, the risk factor increases after the age of 65.
- **Sex**- It appears that women have a higher risk of developing Alzheimer's then men, mainly because women tend to live longer.
- **Past head trauma**- Patients who have experienced severe head trauma appear to have a greater risk in developing Alzheimer's disease.
- **Lifestyle**- Although, there have been no definitive risk factors associated with life syle habits and Alzheimer's, there are some risk factors which may suggest a higher risk of developing

Alzheimer's disease along with heart disease. Some of these factors include:

- Smoking or second hand smoking
- Obestiy
- Lack of exercise
- High blood pressure (Hypertension)
- High blood cholesterol (Hypercholesterolemia)
- Poor diet (especiallly the lack of fresh fruit and vegetables)
- Poorly controlled diebetes (type 2 diabetes)

It should also be noted that the as Alzheimer's disease progresses, especially during the last stages, physical functions, such as swallowing, bowel and bladder control, and balance will be greatly affected.

Symptoms- A person who is experiencing the beginning phase of Alzheimer's disease experience forgetfullness or confusion (mild). However, as the disease progresses, the symptoms worsen. It shpuld be noted that the rate in which the symptoms worsen vary from person to person. Let's begin to explore some of the symptoms.

- **Memory**- Patients with Alzheimer's disease, over time, experience memory loss. The disease not only will persist but worsens affecting their ability to perform normal functions at home and at work. Some patients may experience the following:

  - Forget conversations, appointments or events
  - Repeat statements over and over
  - Often misplacing possessions for example, place keys in the refrigerator or money inside a paper towel roll
  - Becoming lost in familiar places
  - Forgetting the names of family members or objects
  - Difficulty finding th right words, or to express thoughts or take part in a conversations

Performing familiar tasks- Patients with Alzheimer's may experience difficulty in planning or performing routine tasks such as playing a favorite game or planning or cooking a meal. A the disese progresses, they may forget how to dress and bathe themselves.

Making judgements and decisions- As the disease advances, they will have difficulty in making decisions such as not being aware that food is burning on the stove, or when driving a vehicle, they experience making judgement calls such has when to stop the vehicle.

Changes in personality and behavior- Often times, as Alzheimer's disease progresses, the way the patient acts and feels may be affected. They may experience:

- Social withdrawal
- Depression
- Apathy (lack of emotion)
- Mood swings
- Irritability and aggressiveness
- Distrust in others
- Changes in sleeping habits
- Loss of inhibition (for example, undressing in public for no reason)
- Wandering
- Delusions

It should be noted that many of the skills learned early in life, are are amongst the last to be lost as the disease progresses. Some of the skills may include:

- Singing
- Dancing
- Hobbies
- Story telling
- Reading

To learn more about Alzheimer's disease and dementia, go to www.alz. org and click on Alzheimer's and dementia. You will obtain a wealth of information regarding Alzheimer's and dementia.

Amyotrophic Lateral Sclerosis (ALS)- Also known as Lou Gehrig's disease named after the famous baseball player Lou Gehrig, is a progressive neurological disease that affects the motor neurons where the cells gradually break doun and die.

The beginning stages of Amyotrophic Lateral Sclerosis (ALS) generally begins with muscle twitching, slurred speech, or weakness of a limb. As ALS progresses, it affects the muscles needed to move, eat, speak, and breath. Eventually, as the disease progresses, it becommes fatal.

There is no cure for ALS, and scientists are still trying to understand why ALS comes about.

Let's now look at some symptoms associated with ALS.

Early Symptoms of ALS include:

- Tripping and falling
- Difficulty keeping their head up or in a good position
- difficulty walking
- Difficulty performing routine activities
- Slurred speech
- Difficulty swallowing
- Weakness in the legs feet or ankles
- Hand weakness
- Clumsiness
- Muscle cramps
- Twitching of the arms, shoulder, or tongue

For more information about ALS, go to www.alsa.org. Here you will obtain a wealth of information regarding ALS.

Encephalitis- Encephalitis is the inflammation of the brain and often can cause flu like symptoms such as; headache or fever. In some cases, there may be no symptoms at all. The most commmon cause of encephalitis is a viral infection.

There are two types of encephalitis, Primary and secondary encephalitis.

- **Primary encephalitis**- primary encephalitis occurs when a virus infects the brain.
- **Secondary Encephalitis**- Secondary encephalitis occurs when the immmune system fails to react to an infection. Therefore, the immune system not only attacks the infection, it also, accidentally attacks the healthy cells in the brain.

Some common viruses that can cause encephalitis include:

- Mosquito-borne viruses (such as West Nile Virus)
- Herpes simplex virus 1 (HSV 1) which can alos cause cold sores and fever blisters around the mouth.
- Epstein-Barr virus (causes infectious mononucleosis)
- Varicella-Zoster virus (causes chickepox and shingles)

Risk factors- The following are some of the risk factors which can increase the risk of developing encephalitis.

- Weakened immune system- Patients whose immune systems are compromised are at a greater risk of developing encephalitis (such as HIV/AIDS).
- Age- Young children or older adults have a greater chance of developing encephalitis.

Epilespy- Epilepsy is a disorder of the central nervous system, where the brain activity becomes abnormal. In some cases, people with epilepsy, may exhibit symptoms of twitching arms and legs, where others may have a blank stare for a few seconds during the seizure. Seizures fall into to catagories, focal seizure and generalized seizure. Let's examine each one.

- **Focal seizure (without loss of consciousness)**- This type of seizure, results in possible involuntary jerking of the body such as an arm or leg. Also, their emotions, or the way things smell, taste, or feel may be altered. The person my also experience spontaneous sensory symptoms such as, tingling, flashing lights and dizziness. All these symptoms occur without loss of consciousness.
- **Focal seizure (Impaired awareness)**- This type of seizure causes the loss of consciousness or awareness. During this type of seizure the person may stare and they may not respond to their surroundings or they may difficulty with perfoming routine movements such as swallowing or walking.

Generalized seizures- Generalized seizures are seizures that affect all parts of the brain. There are six types. Lets examine each one.

- **Tonic seizure**- This type of seizure causes stiffening of the muscles. The muscles which are most affected are the muscles of the neck, back, arms and legs.
- **Atonic seizure**- This type of seizure causes loss of muscle control which causes the person to fall suddenly.
- **Tonic-clonic seizure**- (grand mal seizure)- This type of seizure can cause body stiffening and shaking, and in some cases can cause the sudden loss of bladder control and biting of the tongue and sudden loss of consciousness.
- **Absence seizure (petit mal seizure)**- This type of seizure often occurs in children. It causes the person to stare or subtlebody movement such as eye blinking. Absence seizures, may also cause brief loss of awareness.
- **Clonic seizure**- This type of seizure causes repeated muscle jerking. Clonic seizures mainly affect the muscles of the face, neck, and arms.

- **Mycoclonic seizure**- This type of seizure comes on sudden with brief twitching of the arms and legs.

Let's now look at some the causes, risk factors, and symptoms associated with epilepsy.

Causes- Some people diagnosed with epilepsy, there is no known reason, however, for others, it may be due to a variety of reasons.

Lets examine some of the causes.

- **Head trauma**- Traumatic head injury such as blunt force trauma to the head can cause epilepsy.
- **Brain conditions**- Brain conditions such as tumor or stroke can cause epilepsy.
- **Infectious disease**- Infectious diseases such as viral encephalitis or AIDS, can cause epilepsy.
- **Developmental disorders**- Disorders such as autism can cause epilepsy.

Risk factors- The following risk factors can increase the risk of epilepsy:

- Head injuries
- Stroke
- Dementia
- Age
- Family history
- Brain infections

Symptoms- The following symptoms of epilepsy include:

- Staring spell
- Temporary confusion
- Loss of consciousness and awareness
- involuntary jerking of the arms and legs

Diagnostic tests- Some of the following invasive and noninvasive diagnotic tests may be performed in diagnosing epilepsy.

- Complete Blood Count (CBC) lavender top tube
- Chemistry panels (SST tube) serum separator tube
- Electroencephalogram (EEG)
- Computerized tomography (CT) scan
- Positron emission tomography (PET) scan
- Magnetic resonance imaging (MRI)

Mengitis- Mengitis is the inflammation of the meninges surrounding the brain and spinal cord. In many cases, meningitis is caused by a viral infection. In other cases meningitis can be caused by a fungal or bacterial infection.

Symptoms- The symptoms of meningitis can develop from a few hours to a few days. The following a some of the s and symptoms of meningitis.

- Severe headache
- Headache with nausea and vomiting
- stiff neck
- High fever (which comes on sudden)
- Seizures
- Confusion
- Sensitivity to light
- Lack of appetite/thirst

Let's now explore some of the various types of meningitis.

Bacterial Meningitis- Bacterial meningitis is when bacteria enters the bloodstream and travels to the brain and the spinal cord. Another way bacterial meningitis can occur, is when bacteria invades the meninges due to sinus or ear infection.

Let's look at some of the most common strains of acute bacterial meningitis.

- **Streptococcus pneumoniae (pneumococcus)**- The most common cause of bacterial meningitis is streptococcus pneumoniae. It often occur in infants, children, and adults. It generally causes pneumonia, sinus and ear infections.
- **Listeria monocytogenes (listeria)**- This type of bacteria found in luncheon meats, hot dogs, and unpasteurized cheese. People who are most susceptable of contracting listeria are pregnant women, older adults, newborns, and people with a weakened immune disease.
- **Neisseria meningococcus**- This type of bacteria is highly contagious which mainly causes an upper respiratory infection and can also cause meningcoccal meningitis when the bacteria enters the bloodstream. This bacteria mainly affects young adults.

Viral meningitis- Viral meningitis, is a group of viruses also known as enteroviruses (viruses which enter the gastrointestinal tract). Viruses such as HIV, and herpes simplex 1 can cause viral meningitis.

Chronic meningitis- Chronic meningitis, is caused by a slow growing organism such as mycobacterium tuberculosis. It invades the membranes and fluid which surrounds the brain.

Muscular Scleroisis (MS)- Muscular sclerosis is a dibilitating disease where the immune system attacks the mylen (protective sheath) that cover the nerve fibers. Eventually, the disease causes the nerves to break down and become permanently damages. The cause of multiple sclerosis is unknown.

For more information about multiple sclerosis, go to: www. nationalmssociety.org. Here you will find a wealth of information about multiple sclerosis.

Symptoms- The symptoms of multiple sclerosis vary from person to person. The symptoms can include:

- Tingeling or pain in parts of the body
- Numbness/weakness in one or more limbs
- Double vision (prolonged)
- Complete or partial loss of vision
- lack of coordination
- Fatigue
- Dizziness
- Slurred speach
- Difficulty with bowl and bladder function

Risk factors- Some risk factors of devloping multiple sclerosis include:

- Family history
- Age (commonly affects people between the ages of 15 and 60)
- Sex (women are twice a likely to deveolp MS than men)
- Smoking

Parkinson's disease- Parkinson's disease is a disorder of the nervous system that affects movement. It is a progressive disorder and develops gradually. The disease, in most cases begins with a tremor in one of the hands (sometime barely noticeable). Although, the cause of Parkinson's disease in unknown, research shows that when the level of dopamine (a chemical messenger) drops, Parkinson's disease develops.

Let's now look at some of the risk factors and symptoms of Parkinson's disease.

Risk factors-

- **Heredity**- The risk factor increases when a close relative has Parkinson's disease.

- **Age**- Parkins disease generally begins around age 60 however, Parkinson's disease can begin in the middle or late life.
- **Sex**- The risk factor of developing Parkinson's disease is greater in men than women.
- **Enviromental exposure**- Over exposure to toxins such as pesticides increases the risk factor of developing Parkinson's disease.

Symptoms- Although symptoms vary from person to person, the early ones are generally mild and in the beginning stages may go unnoticed. Some of the symptoms of Parkinson's disease may include:

- **Rigid muscles**- Stiff muscles may occur causing pain and difficulty with range of motion (ROM).
- **Tremor**- The shaking of a limb, often the hand or fingers especially, when the hand is at rest.
- **Difficulty with speech**- Patients with Parkinson's disease may slur when they speak or they may hesitate to talk. They may also speak quickly or softly.
- **Impaired balance/posture**- Patients may experience difficulty keeping their balance or their posture may become stooped.
- **Slow movement (Bradykinesia)**- As the disease progresses, patients may experience difficulty with peforming regular tasks due to slow movement.

For more detailed information about Parkinson's disease, go to www. parkinson.org.

Diagnostic tests of the nervous system- The following are some of the various diagnostic tests of the nervous system.

- Complete blood count- (CBC) Lavender top tube
- Glucose- (Grey top tube)
- Protein- (serum separator tube SST)
- Potassium- (serum separator tube SST)

- Vitamin B12- (serum separator tube SST)
- Folate levels- (serum separator tube SST)
- Lyme disease- (serum separator tube SST)
- Magnetic resonance imaging (MRI)
- Computed tomography scan- (CT/CAT scan)
- Spinal tap- (lumbar puncture)
- Electroencephalogram (EEG)

Chapter 14

The Endocrine System

In this chapter, we will be introducing the endocrine system. The following will be covered.

- Functions of the various glands of the endocrine system
- Disorders of the endocrine system
- Common diagnostic tests of the endocrine system

The endocrine system includes glands which secrete chemical substances called hormones. The hormones are directly sent in to the bloodstream. (When the glands of the endocrine system fail to work correctly, that part of the body will not work correctly). For example; if the thyroid gland is under performing (hypothyroidism), the patient may gain weight or may lack energy. The following glands make up the endocrine system.

- Hypothalamus
- Thyroid
- Parathyroid
- Pituitry gland
- Adrenal glands
- Pancreas
- Pineal gland
- Reproductive glands (ovaries and testes)

Let's now look into each gland and their responsibility. Let's begin.

- **Hypothalamus**- The hypothalamus is an almond shaped gland
  located below the thalamus and above the pituitary gland. The
  function of the hypothalamus includes:

- Regulating body temperature

ENDOCRINE SYSTEM

ENDOCRINE SYSTEM

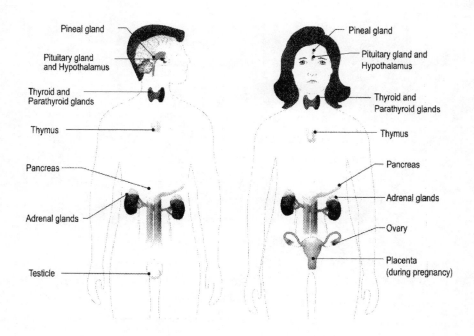

Pineal gland
Pituitary gland and Hypothalamus
Thyroid and Parathyroid glands
Thymus
Pancreas
Adrenal glands
Testicle

Pineal gland
Pituitary gland and Hypothalamus
Thyroid and Parathyroid glands
Thymus
Pancreas
Adrenal glands
Ovary
Placenta (during pregnancy)

- Releasing hormones
- maintaining appitite
- Manages sexual behavior
- Manages emotional respose

The following hormones are produced by the hypothalamus.

- Thyrotropin-releasing hormone (TRH)
- Corticotropin-releasing hormone (CRH)
- Growth hormone-releasing hormone (GHRH)
- Gonadotropin-releasing hormone (GnRH)
- Dopamine
- Somatostatin

Let's now look into each hormone produced by the hypothalamus.

- **Thyrotropin-releasing hormone (TRH)**- The thyrotropin-releasing hormone stimulates the pituitary gland to produce the thyroid stimulating hormone (TSH). The thyroid stimulating hormone stimulates the thyroid gland in producing thyroxin (T4) and triiodothyronine (T3) which stimulates metabolism in nearly every tissue in the body.
- **Corticotropin-releasing hormone- (CRH)**- The role of corticotropin-releasing hormone is the stimulation of the anterior region of the pituitary gland to release adrenocortcotropic hormone (ACTH). The corticotropin-releasing hormone also have an involvement in the body's response to many forms of stress. This includes, emotional stress, physicial stress, internal and external stress.
- **Growth hormone-releasing hormone (GHRH)**- The role of the growth hormone-releasing hormone is to stimulate the pituitary gland in releasing the growth hormone into the bloodstream to stimulate body growth.
- **Gonadotropin-releasing hormone**- The gonadotropin-releasing hormone is secreted in nerves cells in the hypothalamus.

The hormone is released into blood vessels and carried to the pituitary gland which caused the pituitary gland to secrete the follicle stimulating hormone (FSH) and luteinising hormone (LH). Once the hormones are released into the bloodstream, it acts on the testes and ovaries. The follicle stimulating hormone and luteinising hormone also regulate the levels testosterone, oestradoil and progesterone (hormones produced by the testes and ovaries).

- **Dopamine**- Dopamine is a chemical which affects movement, emotions, pleasure, and pain. Dopamine, also has many other roles such as:
  - Memory
  - Movement
  - Behavior
  - Cognition
  - Attention
  - Pleasurable reward
  - Learning
  - Mood
  - Sleep

- **Somatostatin**- Somatostatin is a hormone secreted in the pituitary gland and the pancreas. In the pancreas, somatostatin inhibits the secretion of pancreatic hormones such as insulin and glucagon. Somatostatin also regulates secretion of hormones from the pituitary gland.

Thyroid gland- The thyroid gland is located in the front of the neck just below the Adams apple and wraps around the windpipe (trachea). It's appearance is that of a butterfly because it has wings (lobes). The proper functioning of the thyroid depends of the amount of iodine intake. If the intake of iodine is insufficient, the thyroid could result in a goiter (enlargement of the thyroid) or under performance of the thyroid (hypothyroidism). Excessive intake of iodine can cause the thyroid to produce excessive amounts of thyroxin which can result in the enlargement of the thyroid gland and thyroid cancer.

Disorders of the thyroid gland

- **Hypothyroidism**- Hypothyroidism occurs when the thyroid gland is underactive and is not producing enough hormones. Hypothyroidism can lead to the following symptoms:
  - Constipation
  - Depression
  - Dry Skin
  - Fatigue
  - Problems with memory
  - Sensitivity to cold
  - Slow heart rate (Bradycardia)
  - Weakness
  - Weight gain

- **Hyperthyroidism**- Hyperthyroidism occurs when the thyroid gland is overproducing hormones. Hyperthyroidism, is more common in women then men. Excessive thyroid hormones can lead to the following symptoms:
  - Anxiety
  - Brittle hair and nails
  - Bulging eyes (occurs in Graves disease)
  - Difficulty sleeping
  - Increases sweating
  - Irritability
  - Muscle weakness
  - Nervousness
  - Racing heart (tachycardia)
  - Restlessness
  - Shaking
  - Thin skin
  - Weight loss

- **Hashimoto's disease**- Hashimoto's disease is named after the Japanese surgeon Hakaru Hashimoto. Also known as chronic lymphocytic thyroiditis, Hashimoto's disease is the most common cause of hypothyroidism. It can occur at any age, and mainly affects women. The disease occurs when the immune system slowly attacks and destroys the thyroid gland, causing the gland to lose it's ability to produce hormones. The following symptoms include:
  - Constipation
  - Depression
  - Dry skin/Dry thinning hair
  - Enlarged thyroid (Goiter)
  - Fatigue
  - Heavy/Irregular menstruation
  - Intetolerance to cold
  - Pale/Puffy face
  - Weight gain

- **Graves disease**- Graves disease was named after Robert J. Graves. The disease is an autoimmune disease and leads to overactivity of the thyroid gland (Hyperthyroidism). The disease is hereditary and can occur at any age. The following symptoms of Graves disease include:
  - Anxiety
  - Bulging eyes (including problems with vision)
  - Change in menstual cycle
  - Diarrhea
  - Difficulty sleeping
  - Excessive sweating
  - Fatigue
  - Goiter
  - Hand tremors
  - Irregular/Increased heart rate

- **Goiter-** A goiter is the enlargement of the thyroid gland and is non-cancerous. Goiter occurs when there is a deficiency if iodine in ones diet. Goiter can affect any age, however are more common in women over the age 40. Goiter can also be caused by certain medications, pregnancy, radiation exposure, and genetic risk. Depending on the size of the goiter, the following symptoms can occur.
  - Coughing/Wheezing
  - Difficulty swallowing or breathing
  - Hoarsness (abnormal change in voice)
  - Swelling/Tightness of the neck

- **Thyroid nodules-** Thyroid nodules are growths that form on the thyroid gland. Most thyroid nodules are benign (Non-cancerous). Thyroid nodules are more common in women, however, the risk factors increase with age in both men and women. Most nodules are not normally active. The few that secrete hoemones can cause the following symptoms:
  - Clammy skin
  - Increased appetite
  - Increased heart rate
  - Nervousness
  - Tremors
  - Weight loss

Parathyroid glands- The parathyroid glands are four very tiny glands (about the size of grain of rice) located behind the thyroid in the neck. Their function is to control the body's calcium levels. The parathyroids produce the hormone parathyroid hormone (PTH). The parathyroids help keep the blood calcium levels in a controlled range. For example, when the levels of calcium is too low, PTH is released to bring the calcium levels back to a normal range. If the calcium levels become too high, the parathyroids will stop releasing PTH. Improper balance of calcium can affect the normal functions of the heart, nervous system, and bones.

Pituitary gland- Also know as the Master gland, the pituity gland is located at the base of the brain and is about the size of a pea. The function of the pituitary gland is to stimulate other glands to produce hormones. The pituitary gland is divided into three sections. The anterior lobe, intermediate lobe, and posterior lobe. Let's examine each lobe.

- **Anterior lobe**- The anterior lobe is responsible for body develoment, reproduction, and sexual maturation. The hormones produced also regulate growth and stimulate the following:
  - Adrenal glands
  - Thyroid glands
  - Ovaries
  - Testes

In addition, the anteroir lobe also produces prolaction which causes milk to be produced after the delivery of a newborn.

- **Intermediate Lobe**- The intermediate lobe releases the hormone that stimulates melanocytes (cells that control pigmentation).

- **Posterior lobe**- The posterior lobe is responsible for producing antidiuretic hormones which take back water from the kidneys and save it in the blood stream to prevent dehydration. The posterior lobe is also responsible in the production of oxytocin which aids in uterine contractions during childbirth and the release of milk.

Adrenal glands- The adrenal glands sit on top of each kidney and are divided in to two sections, the adrenal cortex, and adrenal medulla. Let's look at each section.

- **Adrenal Cortex-** The adrenal cortex produces three hormones, glucocorticoids, mineral corticoids, and adrenal andogens. Let's examine them.

- **Glucocorticoids-** In genaral hormones released by glucocorticoids are stress hormones. Hormones released by glucocorticoids include the following:

- **Hydrocorisone-** Hydrocorisone also known as cortisol, regulates how the body changes fats, proteins, and carbohydrates into energy. It also aids in regulating blood pressure and cardiovascular functions.
- Corticosterone- Corticosterone works along with hydrocorisone by supressing inflammatory reactions and regulates immune response.

- **Mineralcorticoids-** The main mineralcorticoid is aldosterone. Aldosterone maintains the proper balance of salt and water as well as maintaining blood pressue.

- **Adrenal androgens-** Adrenal androgens are also referred to as sex hormones or sex steroids. These hormones are released in very small amounts and are generally overpowered by the hormones testosterone and estrogen.

Adrenal medulla- The hormones of the adrenal medulla are released when the sympathetic nervous system is activated also known as the fight or fright response. The hormones secreted are, epinephrine and norepinephrine. Let's look at each of them.

- **Epinephrine-** Epinephrine responds to stressfull situations causing the heart rate to increase and rushing of bloood to the muscles and brain.

- **Norepinephrine**- Norepinephrine works along side with epinephrine. It an cause narrowing o the blood vessels (Vasoconstriction) which can cause high blood pressure.

Pancreas- The pancreas is a gland located behind the stomach and is additionally covered by the small intestine, liver, and gallbladder. The pancreas is both an endocrine and exocrine gland. Lets examine both components.

- **Exocrine**- When food is consumed and enters the stomach, the exocrine cells release pancreatic enzymes to aid in digestion. This is accomplished by release of pancreatc enzymes into small ducts which lead to the pancreatic duct. The pancreatic duct sends pancreatic enzymes along with other secretions also known as pancreatic juices.
- **Endocrine**- Endocrine cells produce hormones that regulate blood sugar. The pancreatic hormones produced are insulin and gluagon and together, they help in maintaining proper balance of sugar in the blood. For insance, insulin lowers blood surgar and glucagon raises blood sugar.

The following are some common disorders of the pancreas.

- **Acute pancreatitis**- Acute pancreatitis occurs when the pancreas is (suddenly attacked), injured by a toxin such as medication or alcohol causing inflammation and damaage to the gland. Other symptoms may include:
  - Abdominal pain
  - Nausea
  - Vomiting
  - Fever
  - Diarrhea

Some of the causes of acute pancreatitis include:

- Hereditary
- Chronic consumption of alcohol
- Trauma
- Infections
- Increased lipid levels
- Medications

- **Chronic Pancreatitis**- Chronic pancreatitis is progressive and ulimately causes destruction of the pancreas and is more common in men. The symptoms of chronic pancreatitis are simular to acute pancreatitis. However, as the disease worsens, the person may develop malnutrition along with weight loss. They may also develop diabetes mellitus as the disease progresses.

Some causes of chronic pancreatitis include:

- Chronic alcohol consumption (most common)
- Hereditary
- Cystic fibrosis

Pancreatic cancer- Reasearchers are still unclear of what causes pancreatic cancer. However, they have found some risk factors which can increase the chances of getting the disease. Let's begin by looking at the some of the risk factors.

Risk factors- The following are risk factors for developing pancreatic cancer:

- Age- 90% of people with pancratic cancer are age 55 and older.
- Gender- Men have a higher risk of developing pancreatic cancer than women. The reason is unknown.
- Smoking
- Obesity
- Diabetes

- Cirrhosis of the liver
- Chronic pancreatitis
- Helicobacter Pylori (H. Pylori)
- Genetics (inherited)

Pineal gland- The pineal gland produces the hormone called melatonin which regulates sleep patterns. Low amounts of melatonin can be due to the following:

- Alzheimer's disease
- Anxiety
- Bipolar disorder
- Seasonal affective disorder

Reproductive glands- Reproductive glands are referred to as gonads or sex glands which produce gametes (sex cells) and sex hormones. In females the cells are the egg cells. In the male the cells are sperm cells.

Female reproductive glands- The hormones which control and make up the female reproductive system are as follows:

- Follicle stimulating hormone (FSH)
- Gonadotropin-releasing hormone (GnRh)
- Human Chorionic Gonadotropin (HCG)
- Luteinizing hormone (LH)
- Oestrogen (Estrogen)
- Progesterone

Let's now look at the hormones which control the female reproductive system.

- **Follicle stimulating hormone (FSH)**- The follicle stimulating hormone is released from the anterior section of the pituitary gland. As FSH flows through the bloodstream and is carried to the ovaries. The follicle stimulating hormone then causes the stimulation of immature eggs (ova) to begin growing.

- **Gonadotropin-releasing hormone (GnRh)**- The gonadotropin-releasing hormone stimulate secretion of luteinizing hormone and follicle stimulaing hormone.
- **Human Chorionic Gonadotropin (HCG)**- The human chorionic gonadotropin is a hormone produced by the placenta. HCG supports the corpus luteum (a mass of cells responsible for production of progesterone) which reinforces the endometrial lining and maintains pregnancy.
- **Luteinizing Hormone (LH)**- The luteinizing hormone is released from the anterior region of the pituitary gland and it's responsibility is to cause the egg to be released from the ovary known as ovulation.
- **Oestrogen (Estrogen)**- Oestrogen, better known as estrogen is secreted by the ovaries and it's function is to stimulate the luteinizing hormone and to stop the production of the follicle stimulating hormone. This is so that only one egg is mature during the menstrual cycle. Other responsibilities of oestrogen include:
  - Secondary sex characteristics
  - Control menstrual periods
  - Control the growth of the uterine lining
  - Bone development by working along with vitamin D.

- **Progesterone**- Progeserone is a hormone which is released by the corpus luteum in the second part of the menstrual cycle after ovulation and prepares the endometrium for possible pregnancy.

Male reproductive hormones- The hormones which control and make up male reproductive system are as follows:

- Follicle stimulating hormone
- Luteinizing hormone
- Testsosterone (main sex hormone)

Let's now look at each hormone indivdually.

- **Follicle stimulating hormone**- in the male reproductive system, FSH stimulates testicular growth which increases the production an androgen-binding protein by steroli cells which are important for testis formation and spermatogenesis (production of mature spematazoa).
- **Luteinizing hormone**- In the male reproductive system, the luteinizing hormone stimulates testosterone production via the interstitial cells of the testes also known as Leydig cells.
- **Testosterone**- Testosterone is the main male sex hormone and it's role is in the development of testes and prostate including the development of the male secondary male sexual characteristics. Other functions include; energy, libido, and sexual function.

Disorders of the endocrine system- Disorders of the endocrine system are broken when down into two catagories. The first catagory is when a gland either produces insufficient amount of hormone (hyposecretion) or the gland produces excess hormone (hypersecretion). The secondary catagory is the development of lesions (tumors of the endocrine system which can lead to overactivity or underavtivity of a hormone.

lead to overactivity or underactivity of a hormone.

The following are some endocrine disorders:

Adrenal disorders-

- **Addison's disease**- Addison's disease is caused by the hyposecretion of hormones of the adrenal glands and can occur at any age and affects both genders. The symptoms may develop slowly and over time. Symptoms may include:
  - Abdominal pain
  - Craving of salt
  - Decreased appetite

- Depression
- Diarrhea
- Fatigue (extreme)
- Hypoglycemia (low blood sugar)
- Hypotension (low blood pressure)
- Irrtiability
- Muscle/Joint pain
- Nausea
- Vomiting (emesis)
- Weight loss

Aldosteronism- Aldosteronism is caused by the overproduction of aldosterone which leads to high blood pressure (hypertension) and can cause the loss of potassium and retension of sodium. Symptoms of aldosteronism include:

- Hypertension (high blood pressure) can be moderate or severe
- Hypokalemia (Low potassium levels)

Cushing syndrome- Cushing syndrome is caused by the high levels of cortisol being produced by the body or the oral intake of corticosteriods. Some symptoms of Cushing syndrome include:

- Acne
- Bone loss
- Fatty deposits (generally around the face (moon face), between the shoulders (buffalo bump)
- Fragile skin (bruises easily)
- Hypertension
- Pink or purple stretch marks on the abdomen, breasts, thighs, and arms.
- Thinning skin
- Type 2 diabetes (on occasion)
- Weight gain

Pancreatic disorders-

- Diabetes mellitus- Diabetes mellitus which also means "sweet urine" is when the body is unable to produce or respond to insulin which results in abnormal metabolism of carbohydrates and also increases the levels of glucose in the blood (hyperglycemia) and elevates sugar levels in the urine.
- Diabetes mellitus type 1- Diabetes mellitus type 1 was once also referred to as juvenile diabetes or inulin-dependent diabetes. It is a condition where the pancreas produces either an insufficient amount of insulin or no insulin at all.

Symptoms of diabetes mellitus include:

- Blurred vision
- Fatigue
- Frequent urination (polyuria)
- Hunger (extreme)
- Increased thirst
- Irritability
- Mood changes
- weight loss (unintended)

- **Diabetes mellitus type 2**- Type 2 diabetes was once referred to as adult-onset diabetes or non-insulin dependent diabetes. Type two diabetes is common in adults and in children with obesity. Type 2 diabetes occurs when not enough insulin is produced to maintain normal sugar levels or when the body rejects the effects of insulin. Symptoms of diabetes mellitus type 2 may include:
    - Blurred vision
    - Fatigue
    - Increased thirst
    - Increased hunger

- Patches of darkened skin (genrally in the armpits or axilary region)
- Sores which heal slowly
- Weight loss

- **Hyperinsulinism**- Hyperinsulinism occurs when high amounts of sugar (glucose) enter the bloodstream. Normal insulin levels are as follows:
  - Fasting <25mlU/L
  - 30 minutes after administration of glucose 30-230 mlU/L
  - 1 hour after administration of glucose 18-276 mlU/L
  - 2 hours after administration of glucose 16-166 ml/UL

Some symptoms of hyperinsulinism may include:

- Craving for sugar
- Difficulty concentrating
- Fatigue
- Hunger (extreme)
- Lack of focus/motivation
- Hyperglycemia- Hypergycemia (high blood sugar) occurs when the levels of blood sugar become elevated. The following symptoms include:

Early symptoms of Hyperglycemia

- Blurred vision
- Fatigue
- Frequent urination (polyuria)
- Increased thirst

Should hyperglycemia be left untreated, ketones can build up in the blood and urine known as ketoacidosis. The following later symptoms of hyperglycemia include:

- Abdominal pain
- Confusion
- Coma
- Dry mouth
- Fruity smelling breath
- Nausea
- Shortness of breath (SOB)
- Vomiting (emesis)
- Weakness

- **Hypoglycemia (low blood sugar)**- Hypoglycemia may occur when a patient skips a meal, takes medications that can increase the insulin levels, or excessive exercising. The following symptoms of hypoglycemia can include:
  - Anxiety
  - Fatigue
  - Hunger
  - Irregular heart rhythm (Arrhythmia)
  - Irritability
  - Pale skin
  - Sweating

Hypoglycemia, can also lead to the following:

- Confusion
- Mental status changes
- Loss of consciousness
- Seizures

Normal glucose levels are as follows:

- Fasting blood sugar 70-99 mg/dl
- Postprandial (two hours after a meal) Less than 140 mg/d

Parathyroid gland disorders-

- **Hyperparathyroidism**- Hyperparathyroidism is caused when over amounts of hormone are released into the bloodstream due to overactivity of the gland. There are two types hyperparathyroidism. Primary and secondary hyperparathyroidism. Lets look at each one.
- **Primary hyperparathyroidism**- Primary hyperparathyroidism occurs when one or more of the parathyroid glands become enlarged which causes the overproduction of hormones resulting in high levels of calcium in the blood (Hypercalcemia).
- **Secondary hyperparathyroidism**- Secondary hyperparathyroidism generally occurs due to another disease which can cause the levels of calcium to drop over time, resulting in the parathyroid hormones to increase.

Symptoms of hyperparathyroidism include:

- Abdominal pain
- Bone/Joint pain
- Depression
- Excessive urination (polyuria)
- Fatigue
- Forgetfullness
- Fragile bones (Osteoporosis)
- Kidney stones (nephrolithiasis)
- Loss of appetite
- Nausea
- Vomiting (emesis)
- Weakness

Pituitary gland disorders- The following are some of the diseases of the Pituitary gland.

- Acomegaly
- Cushings disease

- Diabetes insipidus
- Dwarfism
- Gigantism

Let's now look at some disorders

- **Acromegaly**- Acromegaly is the over production of the growth hormone during adulthood. This hormonal disorder causes the bones of the hands, feet and face to increase in size. Some symptoms of acromegaly include:
  - Enlarged facial features
  - Enlarged hands and feet
  - Enlarged tongue
  - Enlarged organs
  - Deepened voice
  - Increased chest size (barrel chest)
  - Joint pain

- **Cushing's disease**- Cushing's disease is caused by the body receiving high levels of cortisol over time.
- Diabetes insipidus- Although not very common, diabetes insipidus causes an imbalance of water in the body which leads to intense thurst (polydipsia) even after drinking fluids and excessive urination (polyuria). Symptoms (Sx) of diabetes insipidus include:
  - Excessive thirst
  - Nocturia (urination during the night)

- **Dwarfism**- dwarfism is the result of a genetic or medical conditon. One of the causes is the insufficient amount of growth hormone (GH) produced during infancy. The average adult height with dwarfism in 4 feet 10 inches or less. Dwarfism is divided into two catagories; Disproportionate dwarfism and proprotionate dwarfism.

- Disproportionate dwarfism- People with disproportionate dwarfism will have some body parts which are of averagee size and other body parts are small. The most common cause of disproportionate dwarfism is Achondroplasia (without cartilage). Symptoms of disproportionate dwarfism include:
  - Adult height of 4 feet
  - Short arms and legs
  - Short fingers
  - Limited mobilty of the elbows
  - Disproportionately large head

- **Proportionate dwarfism**- Proportionate dwarfism is where all the body parts are small and proprotionate in size. The most common cause of proportionate dwarfism is the insufficient of growth hormone (GH) produced by the pituitary gland during childhood. Symptoms of proportionate dwarfism included:
  - The growth rate is slower than average
  - Height below standard
  - Delayed or lack of sexual development during teenager years

- **Gigantism**- Gigantism is a condition where the pitutitary gland over produces the growth hormone (GH). The conditon is rare and occurs during childhood years. In most cases, the cause is a benign (non-cancerous) pituitary gland tumor. Some common symptoms (Sx) of gigantism include:
  - Increased height
  - Enlarged forehead and jaw
  - Enlarged tongue, nose, and lips
  - Enlargement of the hands and feet
  - Males develop a deepened voice
  - Delay in puberty

Diagnostic tests of the endocrine system - The following are some various lab tests of the endocrine system.

- Adrinocortiotropic hormone (ACTH) – SST tube
- Aldosterone (SST tube)
- Antidiuretic hormone (ADH)- SST tube
- Cortisol (SST tube)
- Calcuim (SST tube)
- Estrogen (SST tube)
- Follicle stimulating hormone (FSH)- SST tube
- Free T3 and total T3 (SST tube)
- Free T4 (SST tube)
- Growth hormone (GH)- SST tube
- Insuline levels (SST tube)
- Luteinizing hormone (LH) SST tube
- Progesterone (SST tube)
- Prolactin (SST tube)
- Renin (SST tube)
- Testosterone (SST tube)
- Thyroid stimulting hormone (TSH) SST tube

It is important, the serum separator tubes be inverted 8-10 times for proper clotting.

Chapter 15

The Digestive System

In this chapter, we will introduce the digestive system. The following will be covered.

- Function of the digestive system
- Structures of the digestive system
- Disorders of the digestive system
- Common diagnostic tests of the digestive system

The role of the digestive is digesting food into small particles which become absorbed into the body and eliminate waste products. Let's now look at the structures and function of the digedtive system. Let's begin

Structures- The structures of the digestive sytem are the:

- Mouth
- Esophagus
- Stomach
- Small intestine
- Pancreas
- Liver
- Gallbladder

- Colon (large intestine)
- Rectum
- Anus

Let's now look at each structure and their function.

Mouth- Digestion begins in the mouth. As food enters the mouth, it is chewed into small pieces. Saliva mixes with the food to start the break down process where the body can absorb and use.

DIGESTIVE SYSTEM

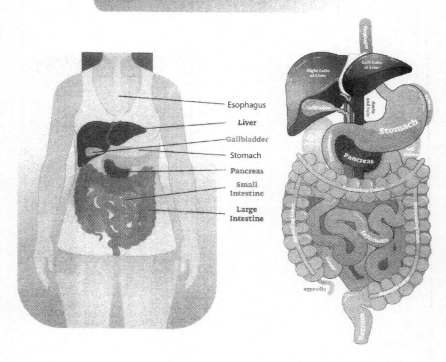

Esophagus- The esophagus is part of the alimentary canal (a part of the digestive tract). It is a muscular tube approximately 8 inches in length and connects the pharynx (throat) with the stomach. The esophagus, also runs behind the trachea (windpipe) and and heart and continues through the diaphragm and into the stomach. At the lower end of the esophagus, a muscular valve called the esophageal sphinchter opens and allows food to enter the stomach. Once food has entered, the valve closes, preventing the contents and acid from moving back up from the stomach.

Stomach- The stomach is a muscular organ located in the left upper quadrant (LUQ) of the abdomen. The stomach is lined with ridges of muscle called rugae which allows the stomach to stretch as well as grip the food. Muscles, begin churning the food and when complete, another valve called the pyloric sphinchter opens and allows the partially digested food from the stomach into the duodenum (the first part of the small instestine.)

Small intestine- The small intestine, also known as the small bowel is approx 20 inches and is divided into three parts; the duodenum (the first part of the small instestine, the jejunum (midsection of the small intestine), and the Ilium (third part of the small intestine). The main role of the small intestine is to absorb most of the nutrients from the food or liquid.

Pancreas- The pancreas is a spongy organ located behind the stomach. It's length is approximately 6 to 10 inches in length. It's role is converting food into fuel for the body's cells. The pancreas has two functions; exocrine and endocrine. As an exocrine function, it aids in digestion by releasing digestive enzymes into the small intestine. As an endocrine, it function is to regulate blood sugar by secreting glucagon and insulin.

Liver- The liver is a reddish-brown colored organ. The liver is located on the upper right quadrant (RUQ) of the abdomen and is protected by the ribcage. The liver is divided into right and left labe and it has many functions, however, it's main function is filtering blood from the digestive tract before it enters the rest of the body. Another function of the liver is detoxifying chemicles and metabolizes (breaks down) drugs. Some other functions of the liver include; secretion of bile (a greenish-brown fluid) which aids in digestion, makes proteins important for clotting.

Gallbladder- The gallbladder, lies beneath the liver and it's primary function is to store bile. When food enters the small intestine, bile is secreted and released through the common bile duct. Bile aisd in the digestive process by breaking down fats including eliminating waste products from the liver.

Colon (large intestine)- The colon (large intestine) is a coiled tube like organ and is approximately five feet in length and is divided into four parts; the ascending colon, transverse colon, descending colon, and sigmoid colon. The role of the colon is to remove water, salt and some nutrients in the form of solid waste (stool) and moves the waste to the rectum.

Rectum- The main role of the rectum is storgage of fecal matter. Fecal matter is stored until full. Once full stretch receptors stimulate the urge to eliminate (defecate).

Anus- The anus is located at the bottom of the rectum and is the last part of the gastrointestinal tract where fecal matter is eliminated from the body.

Disorders of the digestive system- The following are some common disorders of the digestive system.

- Anal fisure
- Appendicitis
- Celiac disease
- Crohn's disease

- Diverticulitis
- Gallstones
- Gastritis
- Gastroesophageal reflux disease (GERD)
- Hemorrhoids
- Hepatitis
- Irritable bowel syndrome (IBS)
- Pancreatitis
- Ulcerative colitis

Let's now look at each disorder.

- **Anal fissure**- Anal fissures are oval shaped tears in the anus. Anal fissures can be cause by strained or hard bowel movements which can cause bleeing or pain during bowel movements.
- Appendicitis- Appendicitis the inflammation of the appendix. Symptoms include:
  - Abdominal bloating
  - Constipation/Diarrhea
  - Loss of appetite
  - Nausea/Vomiting
  - Pain on the right lower quadrant

- **Celiac disease**- Celiac disease is caused by sensitivity to gluten. Ciliac disease damages the finger-like protrusions (Villi) in the small intestines which help in absorbing nutrients from food eaten. Symptoms can include:
  - Abdominal pain
  - Bloating
  - Constipation
  - Diarrhea
  - Vomiting
  - Weight loss

- **Crohn's disease**- Crohn's disease can affect any part of the digestive system. The cause of Crohn's disease in unknown, however, it it thought that family history and genetics may be contributing factor. Some symptoms of Chron's disease include:
  - Abdominal pain
  - diarrhea
  - Rectal bleeding
  - Weight loss

- **Diverticulitis**- Diverticulitis is the inflammation of small pouches called diverticula which form in the weak spots of the digestive system mainly in colon. A symptom of diverticulitis abdominal pain.

- **Gallstones**- Gallstones (Cholelithiasis) are hard deposits formed in the gallbladder. Formtion of gallstones can occur when the gallbladder contains too much cholesterol (Chol) or waste in the bile. When gallstones block the duct from the gallbladder to the intestine, pain can occur in upper right quadrent (RUQ) of the abdomen. Some other symptoms of cholelithiasis include:
  - Diarrhea
  - Irregular stool color
  - Jaundice
  - Nausea
  - Vomiting

- **Gastritis**- Gastritis is the inflammation of the stomach. Gastritis can be cause by:
  - Alcohol (excessive use)
  - Helicobacter Pylori (h.Pylori)
  - Medications (such as asprin or anti-inflammatory medications)
  - Stress
  - Vomiting (chronic)

Symptoms of gastritis include:

- Abdominal pain
- Abdominal bloating
- Burning sensation afer a meal of at night
- Indigestion
- Loss of appetite

- **Gastroesophageal reflux** (GERD)- Gastroesophageal also known as acid reflux is when the stomach acids back up into the esophagus after a meal or even at night.

- **Hemorrhoids**- Hemorrhoids are the inflammation of the blood vessels in the walls of the rectum. Hemorrhoids can be caused by:
  - Chronic constipation
  - Diarrhea
  - Straining during bowel movement

- **Irritable bowel syndrome** (IBS)- Irritable bowel syndrome (IBS) is a disorder which afffects the large intestine. The cause of irritable bowel syndrome is unknown. Some symptoms include:
  - Abdominal pain
  - Bloatng
  - Constipation
  - Cramping
  - Diarrhea
  - Excessive gas

- **Hepatitis A**- Hepatitis A is genarally transmitted by person to person contact such as contaminated water or food.

- Ulcerative colitis- Ulcerative colitis is an inflammatory bowel disease (IBD) which affects the inner lining of the large intestine and causes inflammation and ulcers (sores) in the digestive tract. The cause of ulcerative colitis is unknown. Some symptoms include:

- Abdominal pain
- Cramping
- Diarrhea (some cases with blood in the stool)
- Fatigue
- Rectal bleeding (in some cases, blood in stool)
- Rectal pain
- Weight loss

Common diagnostc tests of the digestive system:

Non-blood tests:

- Fecal occult blood (guaiac test)- A fecal occult blood is used to detect the presence of blood in the stool. The patient is given three cards each one to be used at separate times. The patient should be instructed on how to place the specimen on the cards and then send them back to the lab. The patient should also be instructed to avoid foods which can cause a false positive. Some of these foods include:
  - Raw meat
  - Raw fruits and vegetables (broccoli, cauliflower, radishes, and melons)
  - Foods enriched with vitamin C

- Helicobacter Pylori (H. Pylori)- This test is used to detect the presence of the H. Pylori bacteria that grows in the digestive tract by collecting a stool sample and sending it to the lab for testing.
- Ova & Parasites (O & P)- This test detects the presense of parasites in the gastrointestinal tract (GI tract).

- Stool culture- Stool cultures are collected to test for the presence of bacteria in the digestive tract. Generally, a small sample is collected and sent to the lab for testing. Depending on the lab, results are ready with 48 hours.

Blood tests:

- Amylase (SST tube)
- Bilirubin (SST tube)
- Carotene (SST tube)
- Complete Blood Count (CBC)- (lavender top tube)
- Glucose (Grey top tube or SST tube)
- Glucose tolerance test (GTT)- (Grey top tube)
- Lipase (SST tube)

Note: Always, remember to use proper order of draw and tube inversions.

Chapter 16

The Urinary System

In this chapter, we will introduce the urinary system. The following will be covered.

- Function of the urinary system
- Structures of the urinary system
- Disorders of the urinary system
- Common diagnostic tests of the urinary system

Function of the urinary system:

The function of the urinary system also known as the renal system is to filter waste (e.g., uric acid and urea) from the blood and eliminate it from body as urine. The urinary system also regulates the balance of electrolytes such as potassium (K+) sodium (Na), and calcium (Ca). In addition to electrolyte balance, the urinary system controls blood volume and water content as wll as regulate blood pH.

Structures of the urinary system:

The structures of the urinary system include:

- Kidneys (2)
- ureters (2)

- Bladder (1)
- Urethra (1)

Let's now look at each structure and their function.

- Kidneys- The kidneys are located in the back (posterior) part of the abdominal cavity and their shape is that of a kidney bean. The function of the kidney is to regulate electrolyte balance. Electrolytes are important in maintaining homeostasis (stable conditions) of heart, muscle, and nerve activity. Electrolytes include;

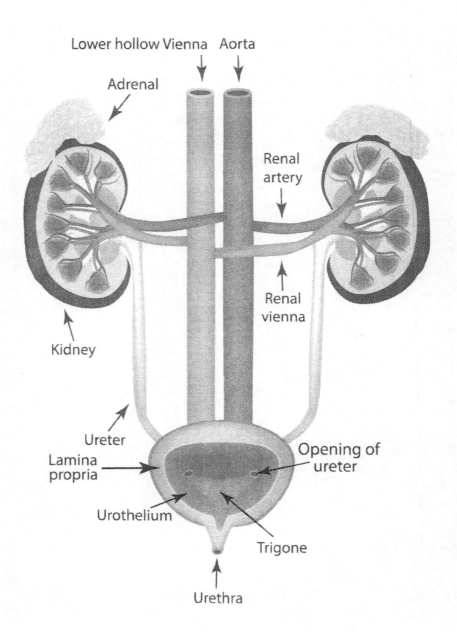

Lower hollow Vienna Aorta

Adrenal

Renal
artery

Renal
vienna

Kidney

Ureter

Lamina
propria

Opening of
ureter

Urothelium

Trigone

Urethra

- Bicarbonate
- Chloride (Cl)
- Potassium (K+)
- Sodium (Na)

Another function of the kidneys is the elimination waste such as urea which is a product of protein metabolism. The kidneys also play a role in the production of many hormones such as erythropoitein which is a hormone that responds when the oxygen (O2) levels in the tissues are low (Hypoxia). Other hormones secreted are calcitrol and renin.

Internal structure of the kidney:

Nephrons:
The kidneys contains over a million microscopic units called nephrons. The function of the nephrons is the separation of ions and tiny molecules and water from the blood, including filtering out toxins and wastes then return any needed molecules needed back to the kidney.

Bowmans capsule:
The bowmans capsule is the saclike structure that surrounds each glomerulus. It is here where the process of filtration begins.

Glomerulus:
The glomerulus are tiny capillaries within the Bowmans capsule. Here is where water, sodium, potassium, and calcium are reabsorbed into the bloodstream. Any remaining elements are eliminated as urine.

Ureter:
Attached to each kidney is a muscular, narrow tube called the ureter. Each ureter measures approximately 10-12 inches in length (in adults) and its role is to transport urine from the kidney to the urinary bladder.

Urinary Bladder:

The urinary bladder is a muscular organ. It is located in the anterior (front) section of the pelvic cavity. Its role is to collect the urine from each ureter and store the urine until urination (voiding).

Urethra:

The urethra is the tube that connects the urinary bladder to the urinary meatus (opening of the urethra) where urine is expelled from the body. In males, the urethra is approximately 8 inches in length and acts as an exit for urine and semen during ejaculation. In women, the urethra is approximately 2 inches in length and its purpose is for urination only.

Disorders of the urinary system: The following are some disorders of the urinary system.

Cystitis: Cystitis is the inflammation of the bladder and in most cases is caused by a bacterial infection. Symptoms of cystitis can include:

- Constant urge to urinate
- Burning sensation during urination
- Blood in the urine (Hematuria)
- Cloudy or strong-smelling urine
- Pressure in the lower abdomen
- Pelvic discomfort

Kidney stones: Kidney stones (renal lithiasis or nephrolithiasis) are deposits made up of minerand salts. Stones form when the urine becomes concentrated causing the minerals to crystalize and band together. In some cases, people with kidney stones may not experience any symptoms until the stone passes through the ureter or moves around within the kidney.

Types of kidney stones: There are various types of kidney stones. Let's explore each of them.

- Calcium stones- Calcium stones are mostly formed in calcium oxalate which is found in food and is made by the liver. Some calcium stones can also be in the form of calcium phosphate.
- Cystine stones- Cystine stones occur in patints with an hereditary disorder that causes the kidneys to excrete too much amino acids (cystinuria)
- Struvite stones- Struvite stones are formed during a infection such as a urinary tract infection (UTI). These type of stones tend to grow large and quickly many times without symptoms.
- Uric acid stones- Uric acid stones can form when there is insufficient amount of fluid intake or when a person has gout ot is losing too much fluid.

Symptoms of kidney stones can include:

- Painful urination (dysuria)
- Frequent urination (polyuria)
- Low urine output (oliguria)
- Red or brown urine
- Foul smelling urine
- Cloudy urine
- Pain which radiates from the lower abdomen and groin

Nephritis: Nephritis is the inflammation of the kidneys which can be caused by infections ans toxins.

Symptoms of nephritis include:

- Cloudy urine
- Pelvic pain
- Frequent urination (polyuria)
- Painful or burning sensation during urination (dysuria)
- Blood in the urine

Renal Failure (acute): Acute renal failure occurs when the kidneys are unable to filter waste products from the blood which causes the levels of waste to increase.

Symptmoms of acute renal failure include:

- Fluid retention
- Decreased urine output
- Shortness of breath (SOB)
- Fatigue
- Confusion
- Weakness

Uremia: Uremia is a condition where the kidneys fail to filter out toxins such as creatinine and urea along with other bodily waste, causing the toxins to end up in the bloodstream. Uremia is a serious condition and if left untreated, can be life-theatening. By the time most patients have developed uremia, their kidneys are damaged, and in most cases, their main source of treatment is dialysis. The procedure to remove the toxins and waste products from the bloodstream is called hemodialysis.

Symptoms of uremia include:

- Loss of or little appetite
- Headache
- Nausea/Vomiting
- Lethargy (fatigue)
- Leg cramps

Urinary tract infection (UTI): Urinary tract infections (UTI) are caused by bacterial infections that enter the urinary tract via the urethra and spreads to the bladder. Although, men are prone to develop a UTI, women have a greater risk of developing a UTI. This is because anatomically, the female urethra is shorter than the male urethra therefore, the distance for bacteria to reach the bladder is shortened.

Common symptoms of a UTI:

- Cloudy urine
- Strong-smelling urine
- Burning during urination (dysuria)
- Constant urge to urinate (void)
- small amounts of blood in the urine (hematuria)
- Pelvic pain

- Note: Parients complaining of any of the above symptoms, you should collect a urine sample prior to the patient visiting their healthcare provider.

Common diagnostic tests of the urinary system:

- Urine culture and sensitivity (C & S)
- Urinalysis (UA)
- Albumin (SST tube)
- Ammonia (green top tube with sodium heparin) This tube must be covered with alumimun foil to prevent light from getting in the tube. Should light get in the tube, it can break down the serum.
- Blood urea nitrogen (BUN) (SST tube)
- Electrolytes (green top tube with heparin or grey top test is **STAT**)

Note: When collecting a urine sample especially for a urine culture and sensitivity (C & S), be sure to use a sterile cup and instruct the patient to avoid placing fingers in cup. Give the patient sterile wipes and instruct the patient to do the following:

Females:

- Wash hands with soap and water.
- Use clean wipes to clean the vulva and perianal areas, starting from the front to back. Repeat the procedure using the second clean wipe.

- With one hand, spread the labia and begin urinating in the toilet.
- With the other hand, place the cup under the genital area and begin catching the specimen in the cup. Be sure the specimen does not touch any skin.
- Avoid over fillling the cup. Half way is suitable.
- Place lid on cup and finish urinating.
- Tighten lid on cup.
- Place cup in designated area
- Wash hands.

Male:

- Wash hands.
- Using a clean wipe, clean the penis from top to base. If the patient is not circumcised, they should pull back the foreskin first. Wtih the second wipe repeat the procedure.
- If necessary, with one hand pull back the foreskin and begin urinating into the toilet with the other hand place cup under the genital and begin catching the specimen. Be sure the specimen does not touch the skin.
- Avoid overfilling the cup. Half way is suitable.
- Place lid on cup and finish urinating.
- Tighten lid on cup.
- Place cup in designated area.
- Wash hands.

Note:
Before handing the specimen cup to the patient, always verify their name and date of birth before placing the label on the container.

Chapter 17

The Skeletal System

In this chapter, we will introduce the skeletal system. The following will be covered.

Function of the skeletal system
Types of bones
Disorders of the skeletal system
Diagnostic tests of the skeletal system

Function of the skeletal system:

At birth, the skeletal system is made up of 270 bones. The number of bones decreases to 206 bones by adulthood due to some of the bones have fused together. It should be noted that approximately 14 percent of body weight is from the bones. Another function of the skeletal system is the storage of calcium and the production of blood cells (hemopoiesis or hematopoiesis) which generally takes place in the bone marrow. The main bones of the skeletal system include:

- Skull- (cranium, mandible **(lower jaw)**, and maxillla **(upper jaw)**)
- Shoulder girdle- Clavicle **(collarbone)**, Scapula **(shoulder blade)**

- Chest- Sternum and ribs
- Spine- Cervical (7 vertibrae), Thoracic (12 vertibrae), Lumbar (5 vertibrae)
- Sacrum- 5 bones fused together
- Coccyx- Small bone at the bottom of the spine
- Pelvic girdle- ilium, ischium, and pubis
- Arm- humerus, radius, and ulna
- Hand- carpals, metacarpals, and phalanges (fingers and toes)
- Leg- Femur, Tibia, and Fibula
- Foot- Tarsals, Metatarsals, and Phalanges

THE HUMAN SKELETON

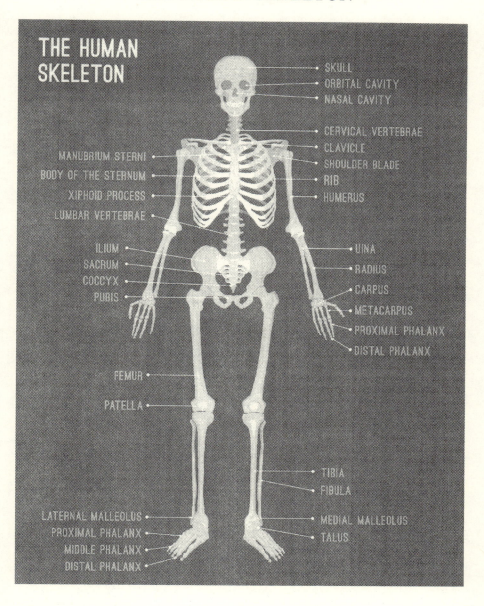

THE HUMAN
SKELETON

SKULL
ORBITAL CAVITY
NASAL CAVITY

CERVICAL VERTEBRAE
CLAVICLE
SHOULDER BLADE
RIB
HUMERUS

MANUBRIUM STERNI
BODY OF THE STERNUM
XIPHOID PROCESS
LUMBAR VERTEBRAE

ILIUM
SACRUM
COCCYX
PUBIS

UINA
RADIUS
CARPUS
METACARPUS
PROXIMAL PHALANX
DISTAL PHALANX

FEMUR

PATELLA

TIBIA
FIBULA

LATERAL MALLEOLUS
PROXIMAL PHALANX
MIDDLE PHALANX
DISTAL PHALANX

MEDIAL MALLEOLUS
TALUS

The skeletal system has six main functions:

- Support
- Movement
- Protection of internal organs
- Blood cell production (hemopoiesis or hematopoiesis)
- Stores calcium
- Enocrine regulation

Types of bones:

The bones of the skeletal system are broken down into five groups.

- Flat bones
- Long bones
- Short bones
- Irregular bones
- Sesamoid bones

Flat bones:

The function of flat bones is to protect internal organs. The following areas have flat bones.

Skull: The skull has a total of 22 bones. Together, they form the cranium which houses the brain.

Flat bones of the skull include:

- Occipital
- Parietal
- Frontal
- Nasal
- Lacrimal
- Vomar

Thoracic cage: The thoracic cage or rib cage consists of 12 pairs of bones. The bone curve from front to back. The upper seven pair of ribs meet at the sternum (Chest). The other five sets of ribs are attached to each other by cartilage.

Pelvis: Pelvic bones are fused together by three bones, the ilium, Ischium, and the pubis. The sacrum has five bones which fuse together at the bottom of the spine. The coccyx (tailbone) make up the rest of the pelvic area

Long bones:
Long bones support weight and bring about movement. Long bones of the lower limbs include:

- Tibia
- Fibula
- Femur (longest bone of the body)
- Metatarsals
- Phalanges (fingers and toes)

Long bones of the upper limbs include:

- Humerus
- Radiu
- Ulna
- Metacarpals
- Phalanges

Short bones:
Short bones are located at the wrist and ankle joints and they aid in stability and some movement. The short bones of the wrist are called carpals, and the short bones on the ankles are called tarsals.

Irregular bones:
Irregular bones are unique, vary in shape and are complex. They are in the Vertebrae and the pelvis. Irrregular bones of the vertebral column protect the spinal cord. The irregular bones of the pelvis protect the pelvic cavity.

Sesamoid bones:

Sesamoid bones protect the tendons from stress and wear and tear. One type of sesamoid bone is the patella (kneecap). Other sesamoid bones are located in the hands and feet.

Disorders of the skeletal system:

- **Arthritis:** Arthritis is the inflammation of the joints. The most common type of arthritis is osteoarthritis followed by rheumatoid arthritis. Let's look at the causes, risk factors, and symptoms.
- **Osteoarthritis:** Osteoarthritis is the wear and tear of the joints cartilage. As damage to the cartilage progresses, the bones begin grinding aagainst each other which causes pain and movement is limited.
- **Rheumatoid Arthritis:** Rheumatoid arthritis is when the body's immune system that attacks the synovial lining of the joints (tough membrane that encloses the joint). As the disorder progresses, it destroys the cartilage and joint within the joint.
- **Symptoms of arthritis:** Symptoms of arthritis include:
  - Decreased range of motion
  - Pain
  - Stiffness
  - Swelling (edema)
  - Redness

Risk factors: Risk factors of arthritis include:

- Age- the risk factor of arthritis increases with age.
- Family history- People who have family members with arthritis have a greater chance of developing arthritis. Family members include siblings and parents.
- Sex- Women are more likely to develop rheumatoid arthritis then men.

- Obesity- Extra body weight can put stress on the joints especiall the knees (Patella).
- Past injuries- People with past injuries such as sports injuries are more likely to develop arthritis in the joint injured.

Bursitis: Bursitis is the inflammation of the bursae which are fluid filled sacs that cushion the bones, tendons, and muscle near the joints. Bursitis mostly affects the shoulder, elbow, and hip. Bursitis can also affect the knees, and heel.

Symptoms of bursitis include:

- Stiffness of the joints
- Pain during movement
- Swelling (edema) or redness at the joint affected

Gout: Gout is the swelling (edema), tenderness, and redness of the joints most commonly in the large toe. Gout occurs when urate crystals (substances usually found in calcium and urate) accumulate in the joint.

Risk factors: Risk factors for gout include:

- **Diet**- Diet rich foods such as meats, seafoods, and alcoholic beverages such as beer increase the risk of developing gout.
- Obesity- Obesity can cause the body to produce more uric acid which can make it difficult for the kidneys to filter out the uric acid.
- **Medications:** Certain medications such as asprin can increase uric acid levels.
- **Medical conditions:** Certain medical conditions such as diabetes or untreated high blood prssure (hypertension) can increase the risk of developing gout.
- **Family history:** Family members with gout can increase the risk factor of developing gout.

Symptoms of gout: Symptoms of gout include:

- Extreme joint pain (especially the large toe)
- Discomfort
- Inflammation
- Redness
- Difficult/limited range of motion

Diagnostic tests of the skeletal system:

- Alkaline phosphatase (ALP) (SST tube)
- Calcium (Ca) (red top tube or green top with lithium heparin)
- Complete blood count (CBC) (lavender top tube)
- Erythrocyte sedimentation rate (ESR) (Lavender top tube)
- Uric acid (SST tube)
- Vitamin D (SST tube)

Chapter 18

The Muscular System

In this chapter, we will be introducing the muscular system. The following will be covered.

The function of the muscular system

Types of muscles
Muscular system disorders/diseases
Muscular system injuries
Diagnostic tests of the muscular system

Function of the muscular system:

The muscular system is comprised of over 600 muscles and their functions are to support the body, maintain posture, body movement (which includes walking, talking, eating), aids in digestion, blood cirulation, and produce heat. The muscular system is broken down into three types of muscles, skeletal, smooth, and cardiac.

Types of muscles:

- **Skeletal Muscle**- Skeletal muscle is a type of striated muscle and functions on voluntary control (works on demand). The muscles are attached to bone by tendons and their main function is to support movement.
- **Smooth Muscle**- Smooth muscles (unstriated muscles) are involunary mucles (Function automatically). The muscles are located in the following organs:
  - Aorta (in the middle layer of the aorta known as tunica media)
  - Bladder
  - Blood vessels (such as arteries and veins)
  - Digestive tract
  - Gastrointestinal tract
  - Iris of the eye

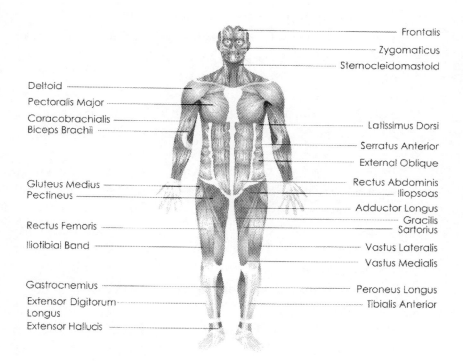

Frontalis
Zygomaticus
Sternocleidomastoid

Deltoid
Pectoralis Major
Coracobrachialis
Biceps Brachii

Latissimus Dorsi
Serratus Anterior
External Oblique

Gluteus Medius
Pectineus

Rectus Abdominis
Iliopsoas
Adductor Longus
Gracilis
Sartorius

Rectus Femoris

Iliotibial Band

Vastus Lateralis
Vastus Medialis

Gastrocnemius
Extensor Digitorum
Longus
Extensor Hallucis

Peroneus Longus
Tibialis Anterior

MUSCLE SYSTEM

MUSCLE SYSTEM

- Prostate
- Reproductive tracts (male and female)
- Stomach
- Trachea (windpipe)
- Ureter
- Uterus

- **Cardiac muscle**- Cardiac muscle is a specialized type of muscle which is only found in the heart (mycardium). Cardiac muscles are made up of muscles which interlock. Cardiac muscle functions uner involuntary control.

- **Muscles of the body**- The muscular system has over 600 muscles. The following are some of the major muscles.

- **Back**- The back is a combination of many muscles which work together. There are five muscle groups. Let's look at each of them.

1. **Latissimus Dorsi**- Latissimus dorsi are the large muscles of the back. These muscles stretch from the sides and behind the arm. Latissimus dori assist in many activities such as pulling or swimming.
2. **Pectorals**- Pectorals are the muscles of the chest. Pectoral muscles are divided into to sections, pectoralis major and pectoralis minor. These type of muscles support the body when stretching or pulling.
3. **Rhomboid**- Rhomboid Rhomboid muscles are located in the upper back. This type of muscle begins at the spinal cord and connect with the scapular bone (shoulder blade). The rhomboid muscle are responsible of all back movements.
4. **Spinal erectors**- Spinal erectors are muscles that help rotate and strengthen the back. These muscles play a role with bending forward and have an active role with posture.

5. **Teres muscle-** Teres muscles are located beneath the latissimus dorsi. This type of muscle works along the the lat' dorsi and the rotator cuff.

6. **Trapezius-** The trapezius is loated between the shoulder and neck. This type of muscle controls movement such as moving the head and neck.

Arms/Shoulders- The following are muscles of the arms and shoulders.

1. **Biceps-** Biceps are located in the front of the upper arm. The are responsiblle for the movement of the shoulder and elbow joints.

2. **Deltoids-** The deltoid muscles are the shoulder muscles. The deltoids are a group of muscle that help with lifting and provide support when carrying objects.

3. **Triceps-** Triceps are located in the backmof the upper arm. Triceps are responsible for stabelizing the shoulder joint and assist with straigthening the elbow joints.

Abdominal muscles

1. **Obliques-** Obliques aid in supporting spine as well as keeping good posture.

2. **Gluteus maxmus-** The gluteus maximus is the largest muscle of the buttocks. It is attached to the pelvis and thigh. They allow the uppper leg mescles to extend and to turn outward.

Leg/Gluteal muscles

1. **Hamstrings-** Hamstrings are the muscles of the upper portion of the thighs. They are responsible for bending the knees (patella) and help move the body forward.

2. **Gluteals-** Gluteals are the largest muscle of the buttocks. Their main rol is to move the legs, maintain balance, walking, and running.

3. **Qudriceps**- The quadriceps are the second largest muscle. The quadriceps are made up of four muscles in the thigh and are located in the upper front portion of the leg.

4. **Gastrocnemius**- Also known as the calf muscles, the gastrocnemius muscles are located in the lower portion of the leg. Their main role is in walking and running.

Muscular disorders- Some disorders of the muscular system include fibromyalgia, multiple sclerosis, muscular dystrophy, myositis, mitochondrial myopathy. Let's now examine each one.

- **Fibromyalgia**- Fibromyalgia is a disorder which causes musculoskeletal pain followed by fatigue, memory, sleep and mood disorders. The cause of fibromyalgia is unkown, however the disorder affects women more than men. Some of the symptoms of fibromyalgia include:

- Fatigue- Often times, the pain from the symptoms of fibromyalgia disrupts the sleep patterns, causing the patient to feel tired even when they feel they had enough sleep.
- Widespread pain- Patients with fibromyalgia complain of constant body ache.

Multiple Scleroisis (MS)- Multiple sclerosis is a disease which affects the brain and spinal cord. The disease eventually deteriorates the nerves causing the nerves to become permanently damaged. Symptoms of multiple sclerosis include:

- Difficulty with bowel and bladder functions
- Dizziness
- Fatigue
- Numbness/weakness of one or more limbs
- Partial or complete loss of vision
- Slurred speech
- Tingeling or pain in parts of the body

Muscular dystrophy- Muscular dystrophy is a progressive weakness and loss of muscle mass. Some of the symptoms of muscular dystrophy may include:

- Difficulty rising from a sitting or laying down position
- Difficulty with running a jumping
- Frequent falls
- Learning disabilities
- Muscle pain and stiffness

Myositis- Myositis is the inflammation of the muscles which move the body. Myositis can be caused by injury or autoimmune disease. Some of the symptoms of myositis may include:

- Difficulty lifting arms or climbing stairs
- Difficulty with swallowing or breathing
- Elevated CPK or aldolase (muscle enzymes)
- Muscle pain which does not get better

Mitochondrial myopathy- Mitochondrial myopathy is a disease which causes both muscular and neurological problems. Some symptoms of mitochondrial myopthy may include:

- Droopy eyelids (ptosis)
- Dementia
- Seizures
- vomiting

Muscular system injuries- There are many types of muscular system injuries such as sprains, strains cramps and tendinitis. Let's look at each one.

- Cramps- A muscle cramp is caused by the sudden involuntary contraction of one or more muscles.

- Strains- A muscle strain is when the muscle of any part of the body is overstretched. Strains can occur if the muscle is overused or misused. Strains most commonly occur in the neck, back, shoulder, and thigh.
- Sprain- A sprain is the stretching and tearing of the ligament. Sprains often occur in the ankles.
- Tendinitis- Tendinitis is the inflammation of the tendon. Tendinitis generally affects the elbows, shoulders, wrist knees and heels.

Diagnostic tests of the muscular system- The following are some of the various diagnostic tests of the muscular system.

- Autoimmune antibodies (lavender top or pink top tube) You should also check with the lab in which you will be working for on which tube they may use.
- Creatinine phosphatase (CPK/CK) (SST tube)
- Lactic acid (Gray top tube with the additive sodium floride or sodium oxalate may be used)
- Lactic dehydrogenase (LD/LDH) (Green top tube with the additive sodium heparin or lithium heparin)

To view more about the diseases of the muscular system go to the muscular Dystrophy Association (MDA), Muscular sclerosos society, and fibromyalgia association. Here you will find a wealth of information.

Chapter 19

The Integumentary System

In this chapter, we will be introducing the integumentary system which consists of the the skin, hair, nails, and exocrine glands. The folowing will be covered.

- Function of the integumentary system
- Structures of the integumentary system
- Disorders of the integumentary system
- Diagnostic tests of the integumentary system

Function of the integumentary system- The integumentary system is made up of the skin, nails, hair, nerves, and glands. It's primary function is to protect the body as well as retain body fluids, elimination of waste, regulate body temperature, and protect the body from disease.

Structures of the integumentary system-

- **Skin-** The skin is the largest organ of the body and it has three layers. They are the epidermis, dermis, and subcutaneous. Let's go over each one.
- **Epidermis-** The epidermis is the outer layer of the skin and provides a waterproof protection.

- **Dermis**- The dermis is the layer beneath the epidermis. It contains hair follicles, connective tissue and sweat glands.
- **Subcutaneous tissue (hypodermis)**- Subcutaneous tussue is the deepest layer of the skin. It contains fat and connective tissue.

The skin also provides the following functions:

- Protection- The skin is the primary source of defense against toxins, and pollutants.
- Absorbtion- The skin is porous which means that approximately 60-64 percent of what is applied to the skin may be absorbed into the bloodstream.
- Excretion- The skin excretes waste by glands that flush out excess minerals and toxins by sweat.

SKIN

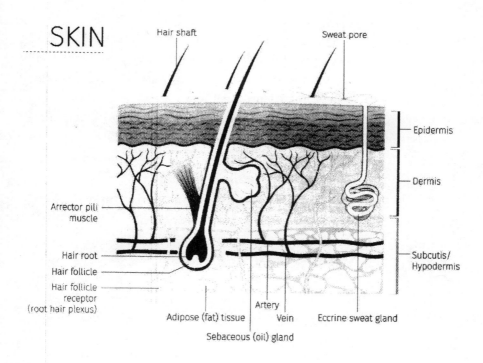

SKIN

Hair shaft

Sweat pore

Epidermis

Dermis

Arrector pili
muscle

Hair root

Hair follicle

Hair follicle
receptor
(root hair plexus)

Subcutis/
Hypodermis

Adipose (fat) tissue

Artery

Vein

Eccrine sweat gland

Sebaceous (oil) gland

- Secretion- The skin secretes from glands beginning at the dermal layer (middle layer of skin). For instance, sweat is secreted by eccrine glands which regulates body temperature. The sebaceous glands secrete sebum which is an oily substance which lubricates and waterproofs the skin and hair.
- Regulation- The skin acts like a termometer. For instance when is hot the brain senses the body temperature rising causing missions of eccrine gland to release sweat causing the body to cool down. On the other hand, when the skin senses cold, it causes shivering making the blood vessels contract helping the body to stay warm.
- Sensation- The skin has four main senses. They are sense of touch, pain, pressure, cold, and warmth. These senses are controlled by the somatosensory system. The following receptors fall within the somatosensory system.
- Mechanoreceptors- Mechanoreceptors respond to mechanical stimuli such as touch and sound.
- Thermoreceptors- Thermoreceptors respond to heat and cold.
- Pain receptors- Pain receptors respond to pain
- Proprioceptors- Proprioceptors receive stimuli from the body and respond to body position and movement.

Nails- The fingernails and toenails are made up of a tough protective protein called alpha-keratin.

Hair- Hair is made up of three layers, the cuticle, cortex, and medulla.

- Cuticle- The cuticle is the outer layer of the hair shaft.
- The cortex is the middle layer of the hair shaft. It provides strength, colour, and texture.
- Medulla- The medulla is he innermost layer of the hair shaft.

Nerves- Nerve receptors of the integumentary system can detect sense of touch, pain, pressure, and temperature. The nerve receptors also work along with the brain, for instance, when the body in getting too close to something hot, the nerve receptors of the integumentary system relay a messege to the brain causing the body to react. The hairs on the skin also aid the receptors to detect temperature and wind change.

Glands of the integumentary system- The integumentary system has four types of glands: Sebaceous glands, sudoriferous glands, mammary glands, and ceruminous glands. Let's look at each of them.

- **Sebaceous glands**- The function of the sebaceous gland is to secrete sebum which is an oily waxy substance. The purpose of sebum is to lubricate and waterproof the skin and hair. When the sebaceous glands become overactive small papules on the forehead, nose, and cheeks may appear. This condition is known as seborrhoea.

- **Sudoriferous glands (sweat glands)**- The function of sudoriferous glands or sweat glands is to control body temperature. Although sweat glands are throughout the body, the majority of these glands are on the forehead, armpit (axillary), palms of the hands, and the soles of the feet.

- **Mammary glands**- The mammary glands are located in the breasts. Both men and women have mammory glands however, in females the glandular tissue develops during puberty with the release of estrogen. The function of the mammary glands in females is lactation (production of milk).

- **Ceruminous glands**- The ceruminous glands work along with the sebaceous glands to produce cerumen (earwax) The main function of cerumen is to protect the ear canal from dust and foreign particles.

Disorders of the integumentary system- The following are some disorders of the integumentary system.

- **Acne**- Acne is an inflammatory disorder of the hair follicle and sebaceous gland and occurs when the hair follicles become blocked with oil andded skin cells causing whiteheads, blackheads, and pimples. Acne generally appears on the forehead, face, chest, and shoulders. Acne is common in teenagers, however people of any age can develop acne.

- **Basal cell carcinoma (skin cancer)**- basal cell carcinoma begins at the besal cell level. Often, it appears as a transparent bump on the skin. Basal cell carcenoma appears often on areas of the skin that is exposed to the sun.

- **Dermatitis (inflammation of the skin)**- Dermatitis is a common skin condition. There are different forms for dermatitis such as atopic dermatitis (eczema), contact dermatitis, and seborrheic dematitis.

- **Atopic dermatitis (eczema)**- Atopic dermatitis appears a a red itchy rash and occurs generally inside the elbows, the front of the neck, and behind the knees.

- **Contact dermatitis**- Contact dermatitis occurs when the body has been in contact with a substance that can irritate the skin or cause an allergic reaction. Some of the substances may include, poison ivy, essential oils, or soap.

- **Seborrheic dermatitis**- Seborrheic dermatitis is a condition that causes red skin, scaly patches and dandruff. Seborrheic dermatitis generally affects the face, back and upper chest.

Herpes- Herpes is a common infection that remains in the body. Although there are two types of herpes, they are both similar. They are herpes simplex virus type one (HSV1) and herpes simplex virus type two (HSV2). Herpes is spread from skin to skin contact such as kissing, oral sex, or vaginal sex. Herpes can be spread even if there are no sores or symptoms.

Impetigo- Impetigo is a skin infection which is contagious. Impetigo generally affects infants and children. The infection appears as red sores around the nose, mouth, face, hands, and feet.

Melanoma- Melanoma is a skin cancer that grows in the melanocytes (cells which produce malanin, the pigment which gives skin color).

Melanoma often appears in areas that have been exposed to ultraviolet rays.

Psoriasis- Psoriasis is a chronic skin condition where the life cycle of the skin cells speed up. Some of the symptoms of psoriasis include:

- Dry cracked skin that may bleed
- Itching/burning
- Red patches of skin with thick silvery scales

Squamous cell carcinoma- Squamous celll carcinoma is a type of cancer that affects the squamous cells (the middle and outer layer of the skin). In most cases, squmous cell carcinoma occurs as a result in over exposure to UV ray from sunlight or tanning beds. Symptoms of squamous cell carcinoma include:

- Flat sore with scaly crust
- firm, red nodule
- Rough scaly patch on lip which may develop into an open sore
- New sore on a old scar

Diagnostic tests of the integumentary system: The following are some common diagnostic tests of the integumentary system.

- Biopsy (Bx)- (shave Bx, Punch Bx, and wedge excision Bx)
- Skin scraping- used to test for fungal infections
- Micobiology cultures
- tissue cultures

Chapter 20

The senses

In this chapter we will introdue the five main senses, the sense of smell (olfaction), taste (gustation), sight (vision), hearing (audition), and touch (somatosensation). The following will be covered:

- Structure of the five main senses
- Disorders of the five main senses

Although, we will be covering the five main senses, there are additional senses. These senses include:

- **Chemoreceptors**- Chemoreceptors, control vomiting (emesis) reflexes. They also aid a portion of the medulla in the brain to detect blood born hormones and drugs.
- Sense of direction- Sense of direction allows the person to know their location and whereabouts.
- **Equilibrioception**- Eqiulibriception allows a person maintain and keep their balance.
- Sense of hunger
- Sense of itch
- Muscle tension
- Sense of pain
- Sense of pressure

- **proprioception**- Proprioceptors allow a person the know the location of a body part such as the position of a limb. It also detects changes in muscle tension.
- **Stretch receptors**- Stretch receptor are found in areas such as the stomach, bladder, gastrointestinal tract, lungs, and blood vessels.
- Sense of temperature
- Sense of thirst
- Sense of time

Now that we have gone over some of the additional senses, let's now cover the five main senses.

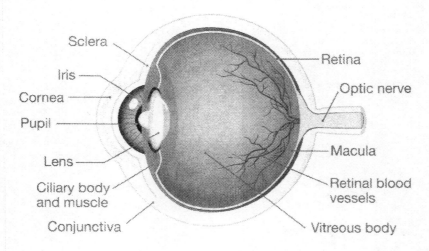

The eye (Sense of sight)- The eye in made up of the following:

- **Cornea**- (the transparent structure which covers the iris and pupil).
- **Aqueous – humor**- (the clear fluid which fills the fron of the eyeball between the lens and cornea).
- **Sclera**- The sclera, also known as the white of the eye, the sclera is the protective layer of the eye which which contains collagen and elastic fiber.
- **Conjunctiva**- The conjunctiva the mucous membrane which covers the front of the eye and lines the inside of the eyelids.
- **Iris**- The iris is the circular structure in the eye. It controlls the diameter and size of the pupil therefore, allows the amount of light reaching the retina. The iris is also the colored portion of the eye.
- **Pupil**- The pupil is located in the center of the iris. It allows light to hit the retina.
- **Lens**- The lens is the transparent (clear) portion of the eye and is located behind the iris. The lens, bend the light rays allowing a clear image in the back of the eye. The lens can change shape for instance, when you want to focus on close objects, the lens becomes fatter and to focus on distant objects the lens becomes thinner.
- **Ciliary body**- The ciliary body connects the iris with the choroid (the thin layer of connective tissue which provides blood supply to the outer layers of the retina. The muscles of the ciliary body control the shape of the lens.

Disorders of the eye: The following are some common disorders of the eye.

- **Amblyopia (lazy eye)**- Amblyopia also known as lazy eye occurs when one eye has poor vision due to inadequate use. This disorder is most common in children.
- **Blepharitis**- Blepharitis, is the inflammation of the eyelid.

- **Cataracts**- Cataracts occur when the lens slowly become opaque causing the vision to become misty or cloudy.
- **Conjunctivitis**- conjunctivitis is the inflammation of the conjunctiva which is the thin transparent layer tissue that covers the inner section of the eyelid and also covers the sclera (white of the eye).
- **Glaucoma**- Glaucoma is caused by the build-up of fluid in the eye causing pressure and eventual damage to the optic nerve.
- **Hyperopia (farsighted)**- Hyperopia also known as farsighted occurs when the eye becomes too short causing the images to focus behind the retina instead of on the retina causing images close up to become blurry.
- **Myopia (nearsighted)**- Myopia also known as nearsighted occurs when light cannot focus on the retina causing objects which are far to appear blurry.
- **Presbyopia**- Presbyopia is an age-related disorder where the eye eventually loses the ability to focus on objects which are close-up.
- **Ptosis**- Ptosis is the drooping of the eyelid

The nose (sense of smell)- The sense of smell is possible because of specialized cells found in the nose. These cells are called olfactory sensory neurons. The nose has approximately 400 odor receptors.

The nose, is made up of cartilage, bone, and muscle. The Shape of the nose is determined by the ethmoid bone and nasal septum (cartilage that divides the nose into right and left. The function of the nose is to warm inhaled air. The hairs in the nose prevent large particles from enytering the lungs. Deep in the nose, there are microscopic hairs called cilia. Cilia move mucous out of the senses and the back of the nose.

Disorders of the nose: The following are some common disorders of the nose.

- **Epistaxis**- Also known as a nosebleed, epistaxis can be spontaneous or due to nose trama.
- **Nasal polyps**- Nasal polyps are benign (noncancerous) growths on the lining of the nasal passages.
- **Rhinitis**- Rhinitis is the inflammation of the musous membrane inside the nose or simply known as inflammation of the nose.
- **Sinusitis**- Sinusitis is the inflammation of the lining of the sinuses

The tongue (sense of taste)- Aside from sense of taste, the tongue has several roles such as, it aids in the movement of food when chewing (mastication) as well as assists in swallowing. Other functions include speech and taste.

The tongue is a muscular organ and is covered by pink mucosa (tissue). The tiny bumps on the tongue which give its rough texture are called papillae.

There are four common tastes, sweet, sour, bitter, and salty. The taste buds and locations are as follows:

- Sweet- Tip of the tongue
- salty- Right and left side of the lower section of the tongue
- Sour- Right and left side of the upper section of the tongue
- Bitter- back of the tongue

Disorders of the tongue- The following are some common disorders of the tongue.

- **Canker sore**- Canker sores or mouth ulcers can occur anywhere in the mouth, but most commonly appear on thee underside of the tongue.

- **Glossitis**- Glossitis is the inflammation of the tongue.
- **Oral thrush (candidiasis)**- Oral thrush (candidiasis) or commonly known as thrush is caused by a yeast infection that causes white bumps to form in the mouth and tongue. Oral thrush most often occurs in infants and toddlers.

The ears (sense of hearing)- The ear is made up of the following:

- **Pinna**- The pinna is the outer portion of the ear with ridged structures. It collects the sounds and moves them to the auditory canal.
- **Auditory canal**- The auditory canal connects with the outer ear (pinna) with the eardrum (tympanic membrane).
- **Eardrum**- When the sounds reach the eardrum (tympanic membrane), it causes vibrations which are sent to the ossicles.
- **Ossicles**- The ossicles include three small bones, the malleus (hammer), incus (anvil), and stapes (stirrup). Once the sounds reach the stirrup (stapes), it vibrates against the oval window.
- **Oval window**- The oval window causes the vibrations to enter a coiled tube called the cochlea.
- **Cochlea**- The cochlea, which contains fluid and resembles a snail, sends vibrations to tiny hairs which are connected to the aauditory nerves.
- **Auditory nerves**- The auditory nerves send messages to the brain where the sounds are interpreted.

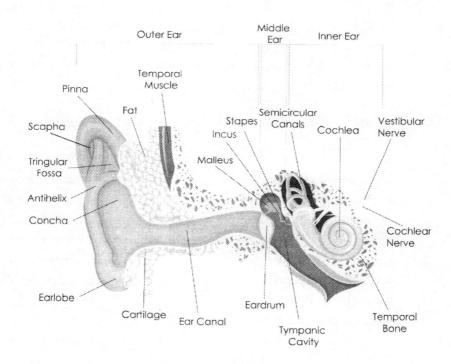

Outer Ear Middle Ear Inner Ear

Pinna

Scapha

Tringular
Fossa

Antihelix

Concha

Earlobe

Temporal
Muscle

Fat

Stapes

Incus

Malleus

Semicircular
Canals

Cochlea

Vestibular
Nerve

Cochlear
Nerve

Temporal
Bone

Cartilage Ear Canal Eardrum Tympanic
Cavity

EAR

EAR

Other parts of the ear include:

- **Ear canal**- The passageway through which sound enters the ear.
- **Eustachian tube**- The eustachian tube connnects the middle ear with the pharynx (throat) and equalizes presssure on both sides of the eardrum (tympanic membrane)
- **Round window**- The round window is located in the inner wall of the middle ear. It compensates for changes in cochlea pressure.
- **Semi-circular canals**- The semi-circular canals contain fluid which help the body stay in balance.

Disorders of the ear- The folllowing are some common disroders of the ear.

- **Cerumen (ear wax)**- Cerumen is produced by glands located in the outer part of the ear canal. The purpose of cerumen is to trap and prevent dust and dirt particles form entering the ear canal. When in cerumen becomes impacted, the patient may complain of ear pain or difficulty hearing. In most cases, the cause of impatation is due to the use of Q-tips which can push the cerumen into the inner ear.
- **Otitis Externa (swimmers ear)**- Otitis externa alsso known as ototis media is the infectiopn of the outer ear canal. Otitis media is often caused by water that remains in the ear usually after swimming which can lead to bacteria growth. Otitis externa affects both childern and adults.
- **Otisis media (inflammation of the inner ear)**- Otitis media is mostly caused by bacterial or viral infections that affect the middle ear. Otitis media can affect both childern and adults.
- **Tinnitus (ring of the ears)**- Tinnitus also known as ringing of the ears is not uncommon. Genarally, tinnitus is an an age related hearing loss condition. The noises heard are phantom noises. The noises can be annoying and can interfere with

concentration. The patient may complain of the following phantom noises associated with tinnitus.

- Buzzing
- Clicking
- Hissing
- Ringing

Sense of touch (somatosensation)- Sense of touch is possible do to many small nerve endings on the dermis (bottom layer of the skin). Sensations of touch, hot, cold, sharp object or soft object are picked up by the dermis, the dermis, then sends the message to the brain for interpretation.

Chapter 21

The Reproductive System

In this chapter, we will introduce the male and female reproductive system. The following will be covered.

- Structures of the male and female reproductive system
- Disorders of the reproductive system
- Diagnostic tests of the reproductive system

Female reproductive system- The female reproductive system have many functions. It produces the egg (ova) for reproduction as well as transport the ova for fertilization.

Structure of the female reproductive system- The female reproductive system is made up of the ovaries, fallopian tubes, uterus, vagina, vulva, mammary glands, and breasts. Let's now look at their function individually.

- **Ovaries**- The ovaries, produce the egg cells called ova or oocytes. Oocytes, are transported to the fallopian tubes where they await for fertilization by sperm. On average, at birth, the female ovaies will contain approximately two milllion eggs. However, approximately ten to eleven thousand eggs will die every month before puberty.

- **Fallopian tubes-** The fallopian also known as uterine tubes are very tiny tubes which carry the egg from the overy to the uterus. The ampulla, which is a portion of the fallopian tube is where the egg is fertilized by the male sperm. Once fertilized, the egg moves to the uterus where it continues to develop until birth.
- **Uterus-** The uterus is a hollow muscular organ. It is located between the bladder and rectum. Once fertilized, the egg (ovum) enters the uterus it inplants itself into the endometrium (lining of the uterus) where it will receive nourishment from blood vessels where it develops into a fetus until time of birth.

HUMAN REPRODUCTIVE SYSTEM

Male Organs

Female Organs

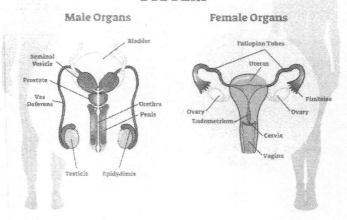

- **Vagina**- The vagina, is a muscular canal which has a soft and flexable lining which provides lubrication and sensation. The function of the vagina is to receive the penis during intercourse, serves a a channel for menstrual flow from the uterus. The vagina is also the birth canal for the new born child during childbirth. A thin mambrane called the hyman surrounds the vaginal opening.
- **Vulva**- The vulva is the outer portion of the female genital. The vulva includes the vagina also referred to as the vesibule the labia majora (outer lips), labia minora (inner lips), and clitoris.
- **Mammory glands/breasts**- The female mammary glands produce milk after childbirth. The breast glands are mainly made up of connective and fatty tissue. As milk is produced, it moves down ducts to the nipples.

Disorders of the female reproductive system: The following are some disorders of the the female reproductive system.

- **Cervical cancer**- Cervical cancer is the growth of tumors on the surface of the cervix.
- **Endomertiosis**- Endomertiosis occurs when tissue which normally lines the the uterus grows outside of the uterus. Some signs of endomertiosis include:
  - Excessive bleeding
  - Painful periods (dysmenorrhea)
  - Pain during intercourse
  - Painful urination (dysuria)
  - Pelvic pain before period

- **Ovarian cyst**- Ovarian cysts are fluid filled sacs which grow on the ovary. Some symptoms include:
  - Abnormal menstuation (metrorrhagia)
  - Irregular periods (oligomenorrhea)
  - Pain during sexual intercourse

Sexually transmitted diseases (STD)- Some sexually transmitted diseases include:

- Chlamydia
- Gonorrhea
- Herpes
- HIV/AIDS
- Trichomoniasis

Uterine cancer- Cancer of the uterus. Some symptoms of uterine cancer include:

- Painful urination (dysuria)
- Pain in the pelvic area
- Pain during sexual intercourse

Male reproductive system- The main purpose of the male reproductive system is to produce, store, and transport sprem into the female reproductive tract.

Structure of the male reproductive tract- The male reproductive tract includes the scrotum, testes, epididymis, spematic cords, seminal vesicles, ejaculatory duct, urethra, prostate, cowpers gland, and penis. Let's go over each one indivudually.

- **Scrotum**- The scrotum is the sac which hangs and stands in the front of the body between the legs. It contains two oval glands called testicles. The smooth muscles which make up the scrotum help regulate the distance of the testes from the body. For instance, when the testes are too warm, the scrotum relaxes, causing the testes to move away from the body. Similarly, when the testes are too cold the scrotum contracts bringing the testes closer to the body.
- **Testicles**- The testicles or testes are the male gonads and their function is produce and sperm. Another function of the testes

is to produce and secrete testosterone which is responsible for fertility, sex drive, and the development of body muscle and bone mass.

- **Spermatic cords**- The spematic cords are a pair of cords within the scrotum. The spermatic cords contain the vas deferens.
- **Epididymis**- The role of the epididymis is to store sperm. Once sperm is produced it from the testes, sperm moves into the epididymis where spem matures before entering the male reproductive system.
- **Seminal vesicles**- The seminal vesicles are a pair of exocrine glands. The role of the seminal vesicles is to produce and store the liquid portion of semen. The liquid produced by the seminal vesicles contains proteins, mucus, alkaline pH which aids in the survival of sperm while in the acidic enviroment of the vagina, and fructose which feeds the spem cells.
- **Ejaculatory duct**- The ejaculatory contains the ducts from the seminal vesicles. As ejaculation occurs, the ejaculatory duct opens, and moves sperm and and secretions from the seminal vesicles into the urethra.
- **Urethra**- Semen passses forn the ejaculatory duct to the urethra. The urethra, which is a muscular organ passes through the prostate gland and ends at the external urethral orifice which is located at the tip of the penis. Urine from the bladder also passs through the urethra.
- **Prostate**- The prostate is a walnut shaped gland which produces a portion of the fluid that makes up semen.
- **Cowpers gland (bilbourethral gland)**- The cowpers gland also know as the bilbourethral glands are a pair of pea- sized exocrine glands. The function of the cowpers glands is to secrete an alkaline fluid into the urethra which lubricates the urethra and neutralizes the acids remaining in the urethra after urination.
- **Penis**- The penis is he male sex organ. Large pockets in the penis fill with blood allowing the penis to become erect. Aside

from expelling semen, the penis also expels urine though the
urethra.

Disorders of the male reproductive system- The following are some
disorders of the male reproductive system.

- **Epididymitis**- Epididymitis is the inflammation of the
  epididymis and it generally caused by a bacterial infection.
  Epididymitis can be acute or chronic.
- **Erectile dysfunction (ED)**- Erectile dysfunction is the inability
  to obtain or maintain an erection.
- **Prostate cancer**- Prostate cancer occurs when the cells of the
  prostate gland develop into tumor cells. During early stages
  of prostate cancer, rher may not be any symptoms. When
  symptoms of prostate cancer do occur the patient may have
  symptoms of:
  - Frequent urination (polyuria)
  - Difficulty mainting a normal stream of urine
  - Blood in the urine (hematuria)
  - Painful urination (dysuria)

- **Sexually transmitted diseases (STD)**- Some sexuallly
  transmitted diseases include:
  - Chlamydia
  - Genital herpes
  - Gonorrhea
  - HIV/AIDS
  - Trichomoniasis

- **Diagnostic tests of the reproductive system**- The following
  are some of common laboratory tests of the male and female
  reproductive system.

Female reproductive system

- Estrogen (SST tube)
- Follicle stimulating hormone (FSH)-(SST tube)
- Human chorionic gonadotropin (HCG)-(SST tube)
- Luteinizing hormone (LH)-(SST tube)
- Mammography (X-ray of the breast)
- Pap smears (test used to detect vaginal or cervical disease)
- Rapid plasma reagin (RPR)-(SST tube)

Male reproductive system

- Prostate specific antigen (PSA)-(SST tube)
- Prostate biopsy
- Rapid plasma reagin (RPR)-(SST tube)
- Testosterone- (SST tube)

Glossary

A

ABO (blood groups)- Blood group system that recognizes the four blood types; A, B, AB, and O.

Additive- A substance such as an anticoagulant or clot activator added in a blood collection tube.

Aerobic- With oxygen.

Agglutination- The process of clumping; such as when antibodies attach to the surface of red blood cells (RBCs) of a different blood type.

Albumin- A plasma protein produced bt the liver.

Alveoli- Sac-like chambers in the lungs where oxygen (O2) and carbon dioxide (CO2) takes place.

Anaerobic- Without oxygen.

Anemia- A deficiency of red blood cells (RBCs) in the blood.

Aneurysm- The weakening of an arterial wall causing a causing a large bulge.

Antecubital Fossa- The elbow region of the arm where the major venipuncture veins ar located.

Antibody- A blood protein produced by the body which fights foreign proteins or antigens.

Anticoagulant- A substance which inhibits blood coagultion (clotting).

Antiseptic- A germicidal which is used to clean skin prior to skin puncture such as (Alcohol or povidone iodine).

Aorta- The largest artery in the body that carries blood from the left ventricle of the heart.

Arrythmia- Abnormal or irregular heart rhythm.

Arteries- Large, thick -walled vessels which take blood away from the heart.

Arterioles- smallest branches of arteries which lead to capillaries.

Arteriosclerosis- Plaque build-up in the arteries causing hardening and loss of elacsticity of the artery walls.

Atherosclerosis- The build-up of lipids (fat) in the arteries.

Atria- Upper chambers of the heart which receive blood from the rest of the body.

B

Basal state- State of the body early in the morning, generally twelve hours after a meal or activity.

Basilic vein- The vein located in the inner side of the antecubital fossa.

Basophils- A type of white blood cell (WBC) which makes up less than 1% of the WBC population.

Bedside manner- The healthcare professionals attitude toward the patient.

Bevel- The slanted portion of the needle which eases needle insertion.

Biohazard- A type of agent or condition which can pose hazerdous conditions.

Bloodborne pathogen- Infectious microorganisms present in human blood which can lead to disease. Such pathogens include but are not limited to, human immmundeficiency virus (the disease which caused AIDS), hepatitis B (HBV).

Blood pressure (BP)- Measures the pressure of blood exerted against the inner walls of the blood vessels.

Brachial artery- The main blood vessel of the upper arm. It is located in the medial anterior section of the antecubital fossa.

Bradycardia- Heart rate less than 60 beats per minute.

Bundle of his- A division of the electrical conduction system of the heart which sends impulses from the atrioventricular node (AV node) to the ventricles of the heart.

Butterfly needle- A short needle ranging from ½ inch to ¾ inch with a thin flexible catheter line attached. Another name for butterfly is winged infusion set.

C

Capillaries- The smallest blood vessels which connect arterioles and venules.

Cardiac cycle- One complete contraction and relaxation of the heart.

Cardiac output- The volumn of blood pumped out by the heart in one minute.

CDC- Centers for disease control and prevention.

Centrifugation- The process of separating substances such as blood or urine by using a centrifuge.

Cephalic vein- located in the lateral aspect of the antecubital fossa. It is the second choice vein for venipuncture.

Certification- The process of providing an official document acknowledging status or level of achievement.

Chain of infection- a sequence of events that lead to infection.

Circulatory system- A system which consists of the heart, blood, and blood, and blood vessels, together, ciculating blood and lymph through the body.

Clean catch- Method used to prevent bacteria collected from the genital area from contaminating a urine sample.

Clot activator- An additive that enhances coagulation (clotting).

Coagulation- The processing of clottting.

Collapsed vein- Result of chronic use of intravenous injections such as drug abuse.

Contact precautions- The use of wearing gloves and gown to prevent the spread of infections or diseases when touching a patient or items.

Crossmatch (x-match)- A blood test used to determine compatibility before a transfusion.

Culture and sensitivity (C&S)- Used to identify the bacteria or yeast causing an infection.

Cyanosis- The bluish discoloration of the skin due to poor circulation or poor oxygenation of blood.

D

Dermis- The thick layer of tissue, below the epidermis. It contains the blood vesssels, lymph vessels, glands, and hair follicles.

Diabetes mellitus- A condition where carbohydrates, fats, and protein metabolism are impaired due to lack of insulin.

Diastolic pressure- The relaxation phase of the cardiac cycle. It is the bottom number when taking a blood pressure.

Differential- determines the percentage and characteristics of each white blood cell (WBC).

Discard tube- Tube with no additive used to collect and discard to prevent contamination of a specimen.

Disinfectant- A solution that destroys bacteria.

Droplet precaution- The use of infection prevention and control in addition to the use of standard precautions.

E

Edema- Build-up of fluid in the tissues.

Electrocardiogram (EKG/ECG)- The recording of electrical impulses produced by the beating heart.

Electolytes (lytes)- Substances that conduct electricity (such as potassium or chloride).

Embolism- The obstruction of a blood vessel by an embolus such a blood clot.

Embolus- Undissolved matter such aas a blood clot circulating in the blood stream.

Empathy- The ability to show emotions and feelling for another person.

Endocardium- The inner most layer of tissue that lines the chambers of the heart.

Epicardium- The outer surface of the heart and the innermost layer of the pericardium.

Epidermis- The outer and thinnest layer of the skin.

Eosinophil- A type of white blood cell (WBC) that fight infections and also play a role in fighting off bacteria and parasites.

F

Fasting- The practice of restraining or reduction of foods with the exception of water for 8-12 hours prior to the collection of a specimen.

Fibrin- A protein subsatnce involved in the clotting of blood.

Fibrinogen- A protein found in plasma which has an important role in clot formation.

Fistula- An artificial joining of an artery and vein.

G

Gauge- The diameter of the lumen of a needle.

Glucose- Blood sugar.

Glucose tolerance test (GTT)- A test used to measure the body's response to glucose (sugar).

Granulocytes- A type of white blood cell (WBC) with granules in their cytoplasm.

Guaiac test- A test used to detect blood in stool.

H

Hematocrit (Hct)- The percentage of red blood cells (RBC) to the total volume of whole blood.

Hemoglobin (Hb/Hgb)- An iron protein found in red blood cells (RBC) which carry oxygen (O2) in the blood stream.

Hemolysis- The destruction of red blood cells (RBC).

Hepatitis- Inflammation of the liver.

Hepatitis B virus- The virus that causes Hepatitis B.

Homeostasis- The state of equalibrium or balance.

Human chorionic gonadotropin (HCG)- The protein produced by the placenta which appears in blood or urine approximately 10 days after conception.

Hyperglycemia- High blood sugar.

Hypoglycemia- Low blood sugar.

I

Immunoglobulins- Antibodies that are released into the blood stream which attack foreign bodies.

Inflammation- Reaction to an injury causing redness or swelling (edema).

Integumentary- Referring to the skin, hair nails and its appendages. It is also known as the largest organ of the body.

Internal respiration- The process where oxygen (O2) leaves the bloodstream and enters the cells, and carbon dioxide (CO2) leaves the cells and enters the blood stream.

Ischemia- Lack of blood supply to the heart muscles.

J

JCAHO- Joint Commission on Accreditation of Healthcare Organizations.

L

Lancet- A sharp sterile device used to puncture the skin to obtain droplets of blood for testing.

Leukemia- An abnormal increase of white blood cells.

Leukopenia- An abnormal decrease of white blood cells in the blood stream.

Lepemic- Excessive amounts of lipids (fat) in the blood.

Lumen- The opening of a blood vessel, tube or needle.

Lymphocyte- The second most numerous of white blood cells.

Lysis- The rupture of red blood cells.

M

Material Safety Data Sheets (MSDS)- Written information on hazardous hazardous products.

Medidan cubital vein- The vein located in the middle of the antecubital fossa.

Megakaryocyte- A large cell formed in bone marrow.

Metabolism- A chemical process in the living organisms needed in order to sustain life.

Midstream collection- Specimen collected during the middle of voiding (urination).

Monocytes- The largest of the leukocytes.

Modes of transmission- The route in which a organism is transmitted from the host to another.

Myocardial infarction- Heart attack due to obstruction of the coronary artery.

Myocardium- he muscle layer of the heart.

N

Needle sheath- Covering of the needle.

Neutrophils- The most numerous of the white blood cells. They contain granules that are fine in texture.

Noninvasive- A procedure that does not involve skin penetration.

Nosocomial- A hospital of place of care for the ill.

Nosocomial infection- An infection contracted in a healthcare institution.

O

Occult blood- Refers to blood in the stool. (also see guaiac test).

Order of draw- A specific order in which tubes are collected to minimize contamination of a specimen due to carryover of an additive between tubes.

OSHA- Occupational Safety and Health Administration.

Ova & Parasite (O&P)- The collection of a stool sample to test for the presence of intestinal parasites.

P

Palpating- The process of touching or feeling for a vein.

Pathogen- A substance or organism capable of causing a disease.

Pathogenic- Capable of causing a disease.

Patient identification- The process of verifying a patients identity.

Patients Bill of Rights- The rights of a patient while in a hospital or healthcare facility.

Pediatric tubes- Small vacutainer tubes used for pediatric patients and patients with small veins.

Pericardial fluid- Fluid that surrounds the pericardial cavity.

Pericardium- The sac which surrounds the heart.

Personal Protective Equipment (PPE)- Consists of protective gear required by OSHA when handeling body fluids. Gear consists of; disposable gloves, lab coat, goggles, or masks.

Phlebitis- Inflammation of a vein.

Phlebotomy- The process of collecting blood from a vein.

Plasma- A clear/pale yellow fluid wich consists of 90% water (H_2O).

Plantar surface- The sole of the foot.

Plateleet adhesion- The process where platlets adhere to the injured site.

Plural fluid- Fluid that surrounds the plural cavity.

Point of care testing (POCT)- Tests performed at the time and place of paient care. (example; UA, rapid strep, rapid HCG test).

Polycytemia- Over-production of red blood cells.

Postprandial- After a meal.

Potassium (K+)- Essential for normal muscle activity and conduction of nerve impulses.

Pre-op- Before surgery.

Professionalism- The qualities that characterizes manners of professional person.

Prothrombin- A protein in the bloood which is involved coagulation (clotting).

Pulmonary circulation- A part of the circulatory system which removes carbon dioxide, and returns oxygenated blood back to the heart.

Pulse- A measurement of pressure put on the ventricles as they contract and blood is forced out of the heart and propelled through the arteries.

Pulse oximeter- A devise used to measure O2 (oxygen) saturation.

Q

Quality assurance- (QA) A program that maintains a level of quality by performing scheduled audits.

Quality control (QC)- A process used to measure the quality of a product.

Quantity not sufficient (QNS)- Insufficient amount of specimen received to process a specimen.

R

Referance values- Normal values for lab tests. (example; the normal fasting blood sugar value is 100-125mg/dl).

Reticulocyte- Immature red blood cells in the blood stream.

Rh antigen- A protein found on the surface of a red blood cell. Blood containing the protein are Rh positive. Blood lacking the protein are Rh negative.

Rh immunoglobulins- A medication given before and shortly after a mother gives birth to an Rh positive baby.

S

Semilunar valves- The valves that control the blood exiting the ventricles of the Heart.

Septicemia- Pathogenic bacteria in the blood.

Serum- The clear/pale yellow fluid that separates out when blood coagulates (clot).

Sexually transmitted diseases (STD's)- Diseases which are generally transmitted by sexual contact (such as; gonorrhea, and genital herpes).

Sharps container- A hard, puncture resistant, leak proof container used to dispose sharp material such as; needles, and lancets.

Sino Atrial node (SA node)- Also known as the hearts natural pacmaker, the SA node is located in the upper right wall of the right atrium. It's role is to produce electrical impulses which initiate heart contractions.

Skin puncture- The use of a lancet to puncture and collecting blood from a finger or the plantar surface of an infant.

Sodium (Na)- An extracellular ion found in the blood. Sodium helps keep fluids in a normal balance.

Sphygmomanometer- The instrument used to read a blood pressure.

Standard precautions- Regulations set by the CDC to help minimize the spread of infection when working with alll body fluids (with the exception of sweat).

Stat- Processing a specimen immediately.

Susceptible host- A person who is at risk of becoming infected.

Syncope- Fainting.

Systolic pressure- The amount of arterial pressure during the contraction of the left ventricle.

T

Test requisition- The form used to order a lab test.

Thrombocytes- Formed elements in the bloodstream also known as platlets.

Thrombocytopenia- Abnormally low amount of thrombocytes.

Thrombocytosis- Over-production of thrombocytes.

Thrombophlebitis- The inflammation of a vein accompanied by a blood clot in one or more veins.

Thrombus- Blood clot.

Transport media- A medium used to transport a specimen.

Tuberculosis- An infectious airborne disease that affects the respiratory system.

Tunica Adventitia- The outer layer of a blood vessel.

Tunica intimia- The innermost layer of a blood vessel.

Tunica Media- the middle layer of a blood vessel.

U

Urinalysis- A lab test which includes physical examination, chemical, and microscopic analysis for the presence of disease.

UTI- Urinary tract infection.

V

Vehicle transmission- The transmission of an infectious microbe to a susceptible host.

Veins- Vessels which carry blood back to the heart.

Vena cava- Largest vein in the body which carries deoxygenated blood back to the heart.

Venipuncture- The insertion of a needle into a vein to obtain blood.

Ventricles- The lower chambers of the heart.

Venules- The smallest veins.

W

Winged infusion (see butterfly needle)